# a juice a day

## 365 juices + smoothies
### for every day of the year

hamlyn

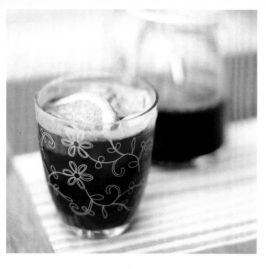
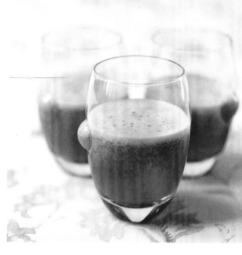
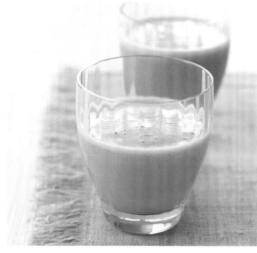
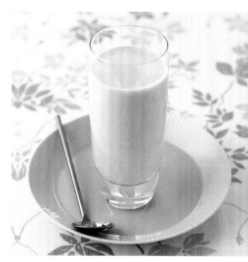
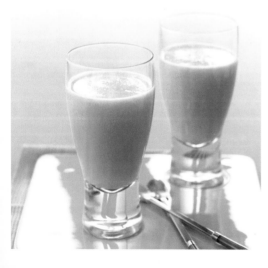
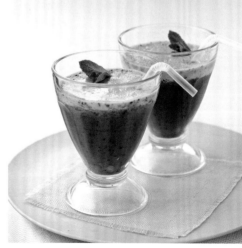

# a juice a day

## 365 juices + smoothies
### for every day of the year

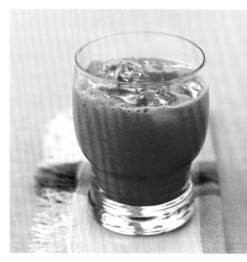

An Hachette UK Company
www.hachette.co.uk

First published in Great Britain in 2017
by Hamlyn, a division of
Octopus Publishing Group Ltd
Carmelite House
50 Victoria Embankment
London EC4Y 0DZ
www.octopusbooks.co.uk

This material was previously published
in *200 Juices and Smoothies* and
*200 Juice Diet Recipes*

Distributed in the US by
Hachette Book Group
1290 Avenue of the Americas
4th and 5th Floors
New York, NY 10020

Distributed in Canada by
Canadian Manda Group
664 Annette St.
Toronto, Ontario, Canada M6S 2C8

ISBN 978 0 600 63457 7

A CIP catalogue record for this book is available
from the British Library.

Printed and bound in China

10 9 8 7 6 5 4 3 2 1

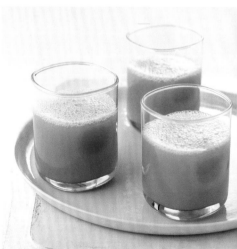

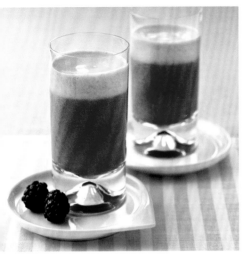

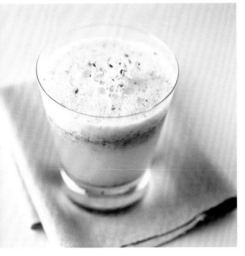

# contents

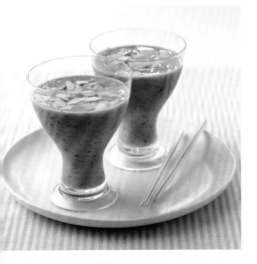

# introduction

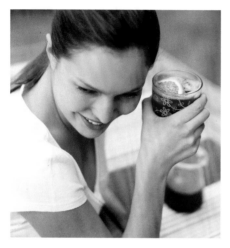

One of the easiest ways to ensure that you have plenty of fruit and vegetables is to include a juice or smoothie in your daily diet.

Lots of important vitamins and minerals are found in the fibrous parts of fruit and vegetables and getting a big hit of those vitamins and minerals would mean eating an enormous amount of food. Juicing releases all the nutrients from those ingredients so that they can be easily absorbed into the bloodstream.

So, what is the difference between making your own juice and buying a carton? The most obvious difference is that the nutrients present in fresh, homemade juice far surpass anything you can buy. This is because bought juice has been pre-squeezed, packaged and usually diluted with water, so that many of the nutrients are lost along the way. There may also be additives in bought juices, including preservatives, whereas at home you can be sure of exactly what you are drinking.

Not only does homemade juice taste better, but the nutrients can be rapidly assimilated into the body. When you begin to drink your own juices you might find that you have a slight headache or are passing water more often – this is part of the detoxification process. Once your body has adjusted to your new regime, the symptoms will fade and you will feel – and look – great.

In this book you will find a daily juice or smoothie for a 365-day year. These include 'next time' recipes, which are either a variation of the previous day's recipe – great if you have leftover ingredients – or a quick 'throw it all in' recipe for when you're in a rush. There are nutritional tips throughout the book, which build upon the following guide to some of the most popular fruit, vegetables and superfoods.

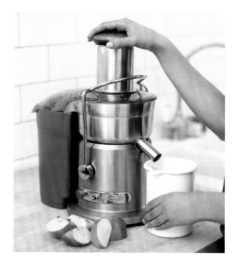

# juicing fruit and vegetables top 40

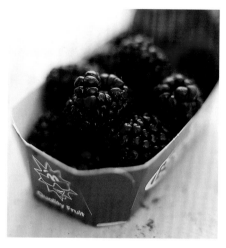

**Apple:** Good source of flavonoid antioxidants that reduce the risk of heart disease.

**Apricot:** Its orange colour signifies good levels of carotenoids, linked with better heart and immune health, and healthy skin.

**Asparagus:** Very rich in folic acid and a really good source of inulin, which boosts levels of friendly gut bacteria.

**Avocado:** Rich in essential fats and vitamin E. Good for healthy cholesterol levels and protecting cells against oxidation (free radical) damage.

**Banana:** Naturally sweet and a good provider of potassium, vitamin B6 and magnesium. Good for boosting energy and maintaining healthy blood pressure.

**Beetroot:** Naturally rich in nitrates, which the body converts into nitric oxide, a chemical that dilates blood vessels and reduces blood pressure.

**Blackcurrant:** Super rich in vitamin C and anthocyanins, linked with healthy skin, arteries and cognitive function.

**Blueberry:** Particularly rich in anthocyanin antioxidant, linked with anti-ageing benefits and improved memory.

**Broccoli:** Rich in folic acid, vitamins A and C and a group of chemicals known as glucosinolates with reported anti-cancer effects.

**Cantaloupe melon:** The orange flesh is a good source of beta carotene and vitamin C. Good for the immune system and skin.

**Carrot:** Rich in beta carotene, an antioxidant that can be turned into vitamin A. Good for the immune system, healthy skin and eyes

**Celery:** Very low in calories and a source of calcium. Good for weight watchers.

**Cherry:** Rich in flavonoid antioxidants. Sour (Montmorency) cherries can help ease exercise-related muscle soreness.

**Courgette:** Good source of potassium and folic acid. Good for looking after your heart.

**Cranberry:** Great source of vitamin C and potassium.

**Cucumber:** Source of vitamin K. Hydrating and very waistline-friendly.

**Fennel:** Good source of fibre and anethole, a substance that's been shown to reduce inflammation. A stomach soother.

**Ginger:** Good for soothing nausea and has anti-inflammatory effects.

**Grape:** Red and black grapes have high levels of anthocyanins for a healthy heart and perkier brain.

**Grapefruit:** Rich in vitamin C and naringenin, a chemical that controls blood sugar and insulin levels.

**Kale:** Rich in vitamins A and C, calcium and iron. Also very rich in the antioxidant lutein, which protects against the eye disease macular degeneration.

**Kiwifruit:** Good source of vitamin C and fibre to give a boost to digestive and immune health.

**Lemon/lime:** High in vitamin C – especially the zest. Also rich in a chemical called limonin, which may have anti-cancer benefits.

**Mango:** Supplies vitamins A, C and E to mop up the free radicals that damage body cells.

**Nectarine/peach:** Both supply vitamin C and some beta carotene (vitamin A) in the yellow flesh.

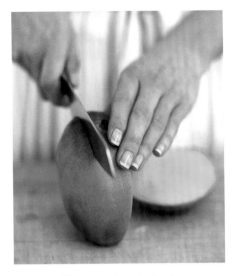

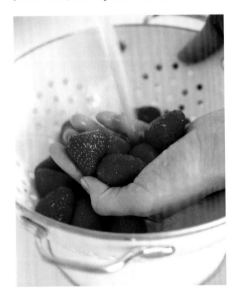

**Orange:** High in vitamin C, plus carotenoid and flavonoid antioxidants that protect cells. Also a good source of folic acid for making red blood cells.

**Papaya:** Rich in vitamin C and beta carotene. Good for the immune system.

**Parsley:** A very rich source of vitamins C and K. Good for your immune system, brain and bones.

**Pear:** Good source of fibre, flavonoids and they have a low impact on blood sugar despite their sweetness.

**Pineapple:** A good source of the mineral managanese, needed for healthy bones and joints, and an enzyme called bromelain that can help digestion.

**Plum:** Red and purple plums are a good source of anthocyanin antioxidant.

**Pomegranate:** Rich in an antioxidant called ellagic acid, which is good for your heart and has anti-cancer and anti-inflammatory properties.

**Raspberry:** A great source of flavonoid antioxidants – good for heart health.

**Red pepper:** Great source of vitamin C and beta carotene. Good for the immune system and skin.

**Spinach:** Great source of vitamins A, C, K, iron and eye-friendly lutein.

**Strawberry:** Rich in vitamin C and anthocyanin antioxidants. Good for skin, heart and cognitive function.

**Sweet potato:** Rich in slow-releasing energy, their yellow flesh supplies vitamins A, C and E.

**Tomato:** A fantastic source of lycopene, linked with lower risk of heart attack, stroke and some cancers.

**Watercress:** A powerhouse of vitamins A, C and E, plus a good source of anaemia-protective iron.

**Watermelon:** Red-fleshed watermelon contains lycopene, which has the potential to reduce the risk of heart attack and stroke.

# key superfoods

**Acai berries:** A reddish, purple fruit from the acai palm tree (a relative of the blueberry), it's usually in powdered form, and provides anti-inflammatory and cell-protective antioxidant benefits.

**Baobab:** This powder is derived from the African baobab fruit, which looks and feels like a velvety version of a coconut and has a huge ORAC value (a laboratory measure of the ability to zap free radicals that damage cells). It's also rich in potassium.

**Cacao:** Better thought of as raw chocolate (it comes straight from the cocoa bean), cacao contains lots of antioxidant and anti-inflammatory phytochemicals, benefitting blood pressure and cognitive function.

**Chia seeds:** Tiny seeds that give 12 per cent of the RDA of calcium and 17 per cent of the RDA of magnesium in a tablespoon. They're also a really good source of omega-3, and turn into a gel when mixed with water, slowing down the release of sugar and stabilizing blood sugar.

**Flax seeds:** Very rich in heart-healthy omega-3, flax seeds add fibre, protein, iron and magnesium to your juice or smoothie. They are also called linseeds.

**Goji berries:** These berries contain vitamin C, vitamin B2, vitamin A, iron, selenium and substances called polysaccharides, which may enhance immune response.

**Matcha:** This powdered green tea is richer in catechin – a type of antioxidant linked to fighting cancer, viruses and heart disease – than other kinds of green tea.

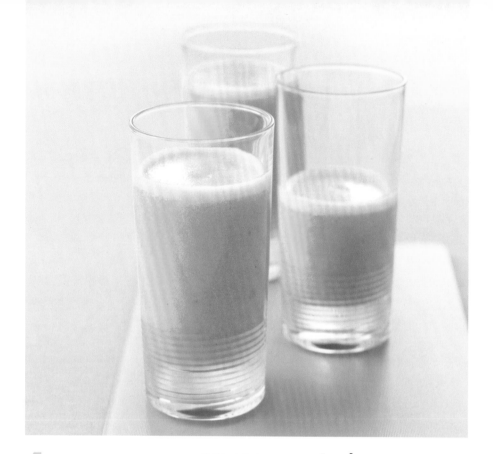

# 1

## orange, carrot + banana
### smoothie

SERVES 1

**1 large carrot**

**1 orange**

**100 g (3½ oz) banana**

**1 fresh or ready-to-eat dried apricot**

**2-3 ice cubes**

Take the top off the carrot and then scrub. Peel the orange. Peel the banana, then roughly chop. If using a fresh apricot, halve and stone; if dried, roughly chop. Juice the carrot and orange together.

Transfer the juice to a blender or smoothie maker, add the banana, fresh or dried apricot and ice cubes and blend briefly. Serve immediately.

## 2

## next time...

Swap the banana for ½ avocado, peeled and stoned, for a creamier alternative.

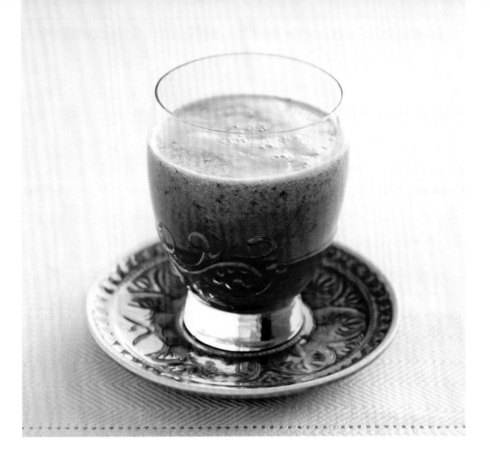

# 3

## blueberry juice

SERVES 1

**½ cucumber**

**1 apple**

**300 g (10½ oz) blueberries**

Trim the cucumber and remove the stalk from the apple.

Juice the cucumber and apple with the blueberries.

Pour the juice into a large glass and serve immediately.

# 4

## next time...

To add some extra oomph to this juice, add 200 g (7 oz) red cabbage, trimmed, to the other ingredients when juicing.

# 5

## blueberry, mango + kefir smoothie

SERVES 1

**1 orange**
**1 mango**
**200 g (7 oz) kefir**
**150 g (5½ oz) blueberries**

Peel and then juice the orange.

Peel and stone the mango, then roughly chop the flesh.

Transfer the orange juice and mango to a blender or smoothie maker, add the kefir and blueberries and blend until smooth. Serve immediately.

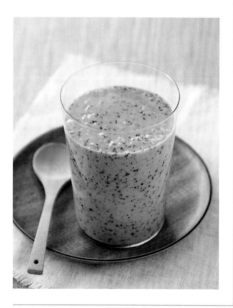

# 6

## carrot + pink grapefruit juice

SERVES 1

**1 pink grapefruit**
**2 apples**
**2 carrots**
**sparkling mineral water,
    for topping up**

Peel the grapefruit, leaving some of the pith on. Remove the stalks from the apples. Take the tops of the carrots and then scrub.

Juice the fruits and carrots together.

Pour the juice into a glass, top up with sparkling mineral water and serve immediately.

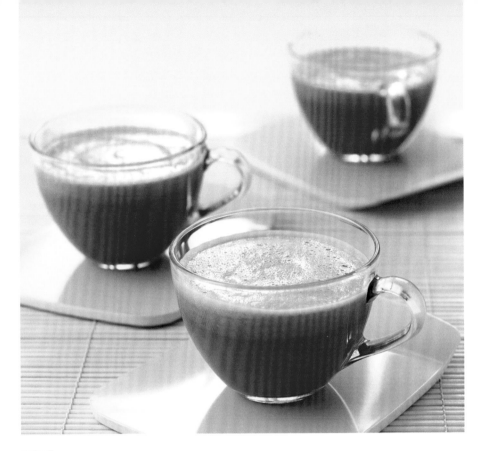

# Tomato, carrot + ginger juice

**2.5-cm (1-inch) piece fresh root ginger**

**100 g (3½ oz) celery**

**300 g (10 oz) tomatoes**

**175 g (6 oz) carrot**

**1 garlic clove**

**2.5-cm (1-inch) piece fresh horseradish**

**2–3 ice cubes**

Peel and roughly chop the ginger. Trim the celery and cut it into 5-cm (2-inch) lengths. Juice the tomatoes, carrot, garlic and horseradish with the ginger and celery.

Transfer the juice to a food processor or blender, add a couple of ice cubes and process briefly.

Pour the juice into a glass and serve immediately.

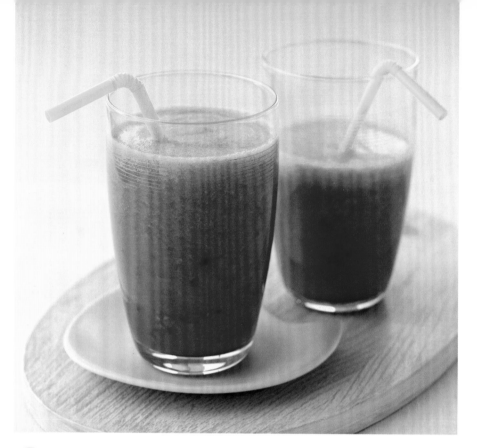

# 8

## raspberry, kiwifruit + grapefruit smoothie

**SERVES 1**

**150 g (5½ oz) grapefruit**

**175 g (6 oz) pineapple**

**50 g (1¾ oz) kiwifruit**

**50 g (1¾ oz) frozen raspberries**

**50 g (1¾ oz) frozen cranberries**

Peel the grapefruit. Cut the skin off the pineapple and remove the core if very tough, then roughly chop the flesh. Peel the kiwifruit.

Juice the grapefruit, pineapple and kiwifruit together. Transfer the juice to a blender or smoothie maker, add the frozen berries and blend until smooth.

# 9

next time...

Blend 150 g (5½ oz) frozen strawberries, 150 ml (5 fl oz) pineapple juice and 150 g (5½ oz) strawberry yogurt together until smooth.

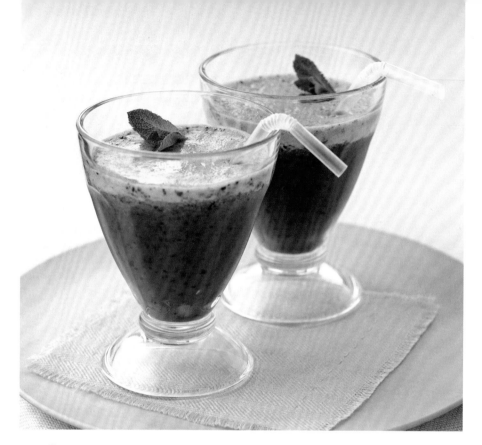

# 10

## blueberry + mint smoothie

SERVES 1

**100 g (3½ oz) frozen blueberries**

**150 ml (5 fl oz) soya milk**

**small bunch of mint, plus extra sprigs to decorate**

Put the blueberries in a blender or smoothie maker and pour in the soya milk. Pull the mint leaves off their stalks and add to the blender or smoothie maker, then blend briefly.

Pour the smoothie into a glass, decorate with mint sprigs and serve immediately.

# 11

## next time...

Process 250 g (9 oz) apples with 125 g (4½ oz) blueberries in a blender or smoothie maker until smooth.

# 12

## red pepper, tomato + carrot juice

SERVES 1

**2 celery sticks**

**1 carrot**

**½ red pepper**

**½ cucumber**

**2 tomatoes**

**25g (1 oz) watercress**

**Tabasco, to taste**

Peel away any stringy bits from the celery. Take the top off the carrot and then scrub. Core and deseed the red pepper. Trim the cucumber.

Juice all the vegetables together, then add Tabasco sauce to taste.

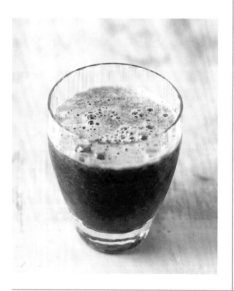

# 13

## banana, mango + coconut shake

SERVES 2

**1 mango**

**1 large banana**

**150 ml (5 fl oz) coconut milk**

**handful of ice cubes**

Peel and stone the mango, then cut it into chunks.

Put the mango and banana in a food processor or blender and process until really smooth.

Add the coconut milk and process again, then add the ice and process until the ice is very crushed and the shake thickens.

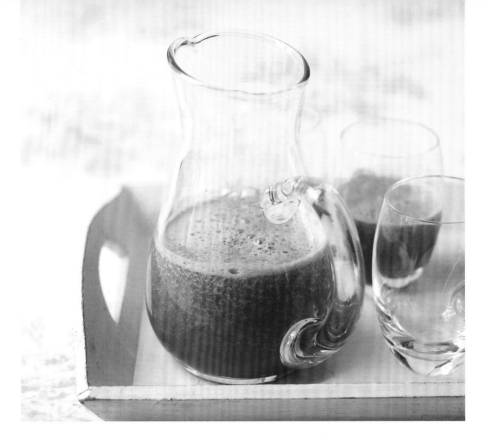

# 14

## three melon + ginger juice

SERVES 1

**100g (3½ oz) watermelon**

**100g (3½ oz) honeydew melon**

**100g (3½ oz) cantaloupe or galia melon**

**2-cm (¾-inch) piece fresh root ginger**

Peel all the melons as close to the skin as possible and deseed. Peel the ginger.

Juice the melon and ginger together.

Alternatively, for a smoothie version, put the melon and ginger, roughly chopped, in a blender or smoothie maker and blend until smooth.

Pour the drink into a glass and serve immediately.

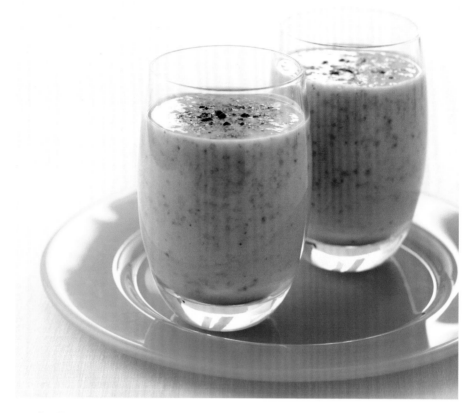

# 15

## strawberry lassi

SERVES 4–6

**400 g (14 oz) strawberries**

**750 ml (26 fl oz) ice-cold water**

**300 g (10½ oz) low-fat live natural yogurt**

**25 g (1 oz) golden caster sugar**

**few drops of rosewater**

**coarsely ground black pepper, to decorate**

Hull the strawberries. Put in a blender or smoothie maker with half the measured water and blend until smooth.

Add the yogurt, sugar, rosewater and the remaining water and blend again until smooth and frothy.

Pour the smoothie into chilled glasses, sprinkle with black pepper and serve immediately.

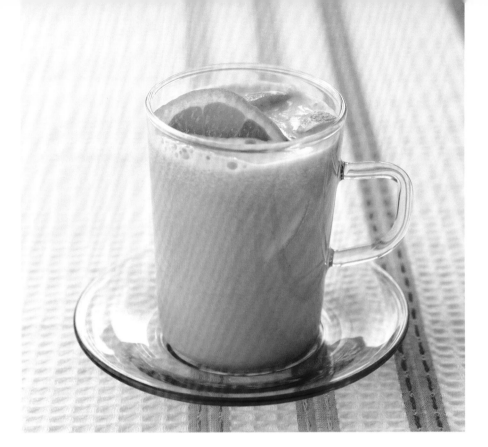

# 16

## celeriac, alfalfa + orange juice

SERVES 1

**100 g (3½ oz) orange, plus extra slices to decorate (optional)**

**100 g (3½ oz) celeriac**

**100 g (3½ oz) alfalfa sprouts**

Peel the orange. Peel the celeriac and cut it into chunks. Rinse the alfalfa sprouts.

Juice all the ingredients together.

Pour the juice into a glass, add orange slices, if liked, and serve immediately.

# 17

## pineapple + pink grapefruit juice

SERVES 1

**250 g (9 oz) pineapple**
**1 pink grapefruit**
**still mineral water, for topping up**

Cut the skin off the pineapple and remove the core if very tough, then roughly chop the flesh.

Juice the pineapple and unpeeled grapefruit together.

Pour the juice into a glass, top up with still mineral water and serve immediately.

 **tip**

Pineapple is great at dissolving the mucus that can accumulate in your system if you have a build-up of toxins.

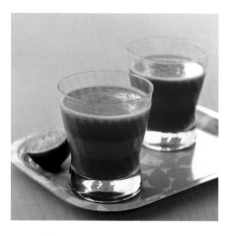

# 18

## papaya, raspberry + grapefruit juice

SERVES 1

**150 g (5½ oz) grapefruit**
**150 g (5½ oz) papaya**
**150 g (5½ oz) raspberries**
**juice of ½ lime, plus extra slices to decorate (optional)**
**2–3 ice cubes (optional)**

Peel the grapefruit. Peel and deseed the papaya.

Juice all the fruits with the lime juice.

Pour the juice into a glass, add the ice cubes, if using, decorate with lime slices, if liked, and serve immediately.

## 19

### gooseberry + orange juice

SERVES 1

**2 oranges**

**100 g (3½ oz) gooseberries**

Peel the oranges. Snip off the tip and flower end of the gooseberries.

Juice the fruits together.

Pour the juice into a glass and serve immediately.

## 20

### carrot, squash + red pepper juice

SERVES 1

**150 g (5½ oz) butternut squash**

**2 carrots**

**1 red pepper**

Peel and deseed the butternut squash, then roughly chop the flesh. Take the tops off the carrots and then scrub. Core and deseed the red pepper.

Juice all the ingredients together.

Pour the juice into a glass and serve immediately.

## 21

### kale + pineapple juice

SERVES 1

**100 g (3½ oz) kale**

**250 g (9 oz) pineapple**

**2 pears**

**½ lime**

Cut any really woody stalks off the kale. Cut the skin off the pineapple and remove the core if very tough, then roughly chop the flesh. Remove the stalks from the pears. Peel the lime half.

Juice all the ingredients together and serve immediately.

**tip**

This juice is rich in vitamins as well as being delicious.

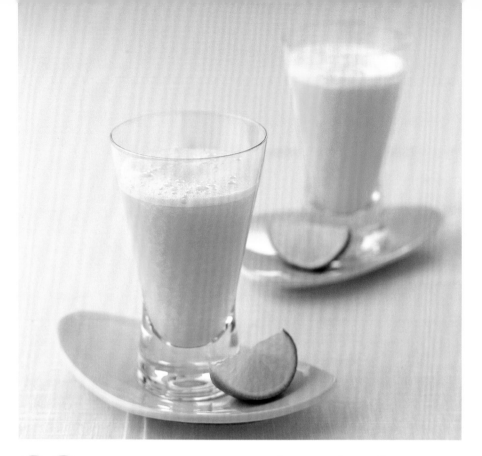

# 22

## mango, pineapple + lime
### smoothie

SERVES 2

**1 mango**

**300 ml (10 fl oz) pineapple juice**

**grated zest and juice of ½ lime**

**lime wedges, to decorate (optional)**

Peel and stone the mango, roughly chop the flesh and put it in a freezerproof container. Freeze for at least 2 hours or overnight.

Transfer the frozen mango to a blender or smoothie maker, add the pineapple juice and lime zest and juice, and blend until smooth.

Pour the smoothie into glasses, decorate with lime wedges, if liked, and serve immediately.

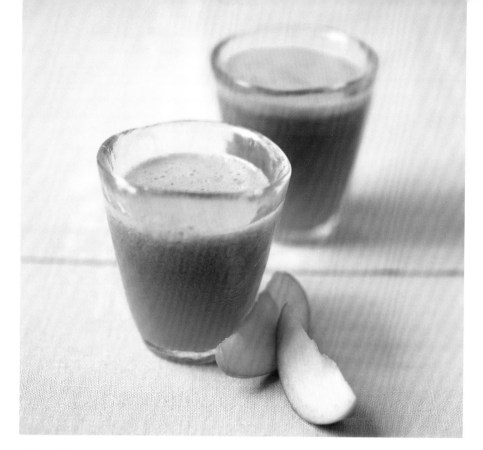

# 23

## green apple, pear + spinach juice

**SERVES 1**

**1 green apple, plus a couple of wedges to decorate**

**1 pear**

**25 g (1 oz) spinach**

**¼ cucumber**

**½ lime**

Remove the stalks from the apple and pear. Rinse the spinach.

Juice the apple and pear together, then the spinach, cucumber and unpeeled lime half.

Pour the juice into a glass, decorate with apple wedges and serve immediately.

# 24

## next time...

Blend a papaya, peeled, deseeded and roughly chopped, and a banana, peeled and roughly chopped, with the juice of 1 orange, 300 ml (10 fl oz) fresh apple juice and some ice cubes until smooth.

## 25

## kiwifruit, melon + passionfruit juice

SERVES 1

**300 g (10½ oz) watermelon**

**2 kiwifruits**

**200 ml (7 fl oz) passionfruit juice**

Peel and deseed the melon and cut the flesh into cubes.

Put the melon in a freezer container and freeze for at least 2 hours or overnight.

Peel and roughly chop the kiwifruits, then put them in a food processor or blender with the melon and passionfruit juice and process until thick. Serve immediately.

## 26

## gingered carrot, orange + barleygrass juice

SERVES 1

**2 carrots**

**2 oranges**

**1 apple**

**2-cm (¾-inch) piece fresh root ginger**

**½ tablespoon barleygrass or wheatgrass powder**

Take the tops off the carrots and then scrub. Peel the oranges. Remove the stalk from the apple. Peel the ginger.

Juice the carrots, oranges and apple with the ginger.

Stir in the barleygrass or wheatgrass powder, then pour into a glass and serve immediately.

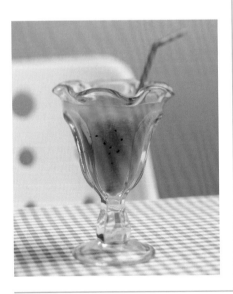

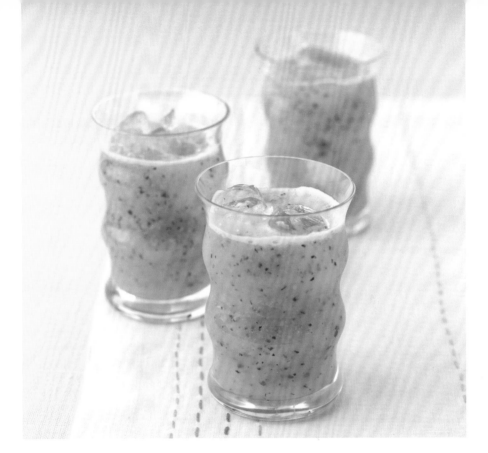

# 27

## mango + mint sherbet

SERVES 4

**3 mangoes**

**4 tablespoons freshly
  squeezed lemon juice**

**1 tablespoon caster sugar**

**12 mint leaves, finely chopped**

**900 ml (32 fl oz) ice-cold water**

**ice cubes**

Peel and stone the mangoes, then roughly chop the flesh.

Put the mangoes in a blender or smoothie maker, add the lemon juice, sugar, mint leaves and measured water and blend until smooth.

Pour the sherbet into glasses over ice cubes and serve immediately.

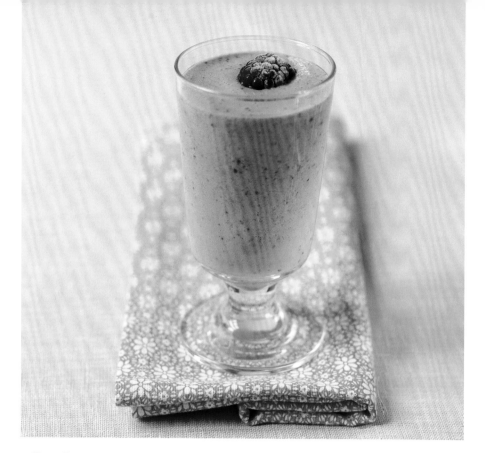

## 28

### mixed berry soya milk
smoothie

SERVES 2

**150 g (5½ oz) frozen mixed summer berries, plus extra to decorate (optional)**

**300 ml (10 fl oz) vanilla soya milk**

**1 teaspoon clear honey**

Put the berries, soya milk and honey in a blender or smoothie maker and blend until smooth.

Pour the smoothie into glasses, decorate with extra berries, if liked, and serve immediately.

## 29

### next time...

Blend 250 g (9 oz) red seedless grapes, 125 g (4½ oz) frozen blueberries and 3 tablespoons fromage frais together until smooth.

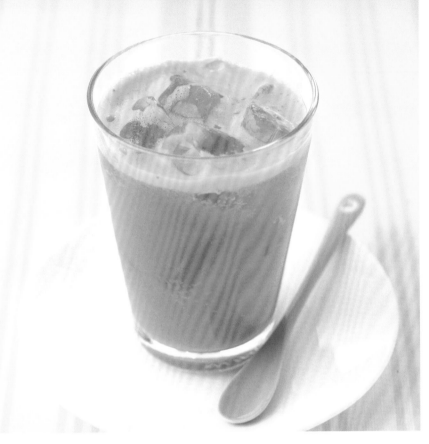

# 30

## banana + fig smoothie

SERVES 1

**1 orange**

**250 g (9 oz) carrots**

**100 g (3½ oz) banana**

**2.5-cm (1-inch) piece fresh root ginger**

**100 g (3½ oz) figs**

**ice cubes**

Peel the orange. Take the tops off the carrots and then scrub. Peel the banana, then roughly chop. Peel the ginger. Remove the stalks from the figs.

Juice the orange, carrots and figs together with the ginger.

Transfer the juice to a blender or smoothie maker, add the banana and some ice cubes and blend until smooth.

Pour the smoothie into a glass, add more ice cubes and serve immediately.

# 31

## apple, cranberry + blueberry juice

SERVES 1

3 apples

150 ml (5 fl oz) unsweetened cranberry
  juice

125 g (4½ oz) fresh or frozen blueberries

1 tablespoon powdered psyllium husks

ice cubes (optional)

Remove the stalks from the apples and
then juice.

Transfer the apple juice to a blender or
food processor, add the cranberry juice,
blueberries and powdered psyllium
husks and blend until smooth.

Pour the juice over ice cubes, if using,
in a glass and serve immediately.

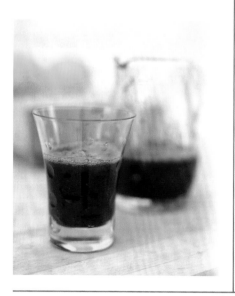

# 32

## tomato, celery + ginger juice

SERVES 1

175 g (6 oz) carrots

100 g (3½ oz) celery, plus extra slivers
  to decorate (optional)

2.5-cm (1-inch) piece fresh root ginger

2.5-cm (1-inch) piece fresh horseradish

1 garlic clove

300 g (10½ oz) tomatoes

ice cubes

Take the tops off the carrots and then
scrub. Peel away any stringy bits from
the celery. Peel the ginger, horseradish
and garlic.

Juice the prepared ingredients with the
tomatoes.

Pour the juice over ice cubes in a glass,
decorate with celery slivers, if liked,
and serve immediately.

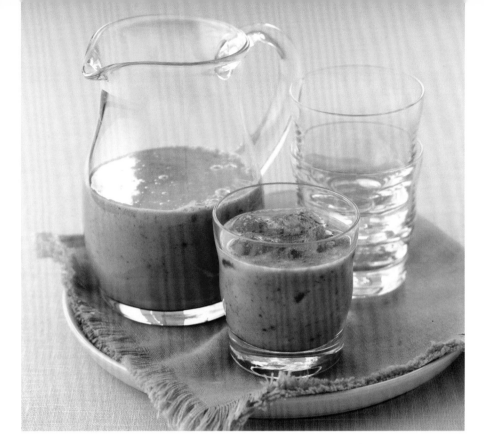

# 33

## prune, apple + cinnamon
### smoothie

SERVES 1

**70 g (2½ oz) pitted prunes**
**pinch of ground cinnamon**
**350 ml (12 fl oz) apple juice**
**3 tablespoons Greek yogurt**
**ice cubes**

Roughly chop the prunes. Put in a large bowl with the cinnamon, then pour over the apple juice, cover and leave to stand overnight.

Transfer the prune and apple juice mixture to a blender or smoothie maker, add the yogurt and blend until smooth. Serve immediately.

# 34

### next time...

Blend a small avocado, peeled and stoned, with 100 ml (3½ fl oz) fresh apple juice until smooth.

## 35

# nectarine + basil juice

SERVES 1

**2 nectarines**

**125 ml (4 fl oz) coconut water**

**1 teaspoon chopped basil (or mint, if preferred)**

**1 teaspoon agave syrup**

**ice cubes**

Halve and stone the nectarines, then juice.

Transfer the juice to a blender or food processor, add the coconut water, basil and agave syrup and blend together.

Pour the juice over ice cubes in a glass and serve immediately.

## 36

# cherry + melon juice

SERVES 1

**300 g (10½ oz) honeydew melon**

**125 g (4½ oz) stoned cherries**

Peel the melon as close to the skin as possible and deseed.

Juice the melon and cherries together.

Pour the juice into a glass and serve immediately.

## 37

# pear, avocado + spinach smoothie

SERVES 1

**1 pear**

**1 apple**

**½ avocado**

**25 g (1 oz) spinach**

**10 g (¼ oz) flat leaf parsley**

Remove the stalks from the pear and apple. Peel and stone the avocado. Rinse the spinach.

Juice the pear, apple, spinach and parsley together.

Transfer the juice to a blender or smoothie maker, add the avocado and blend until smooth.

Pour the smoothie into a glass and serve immediately.

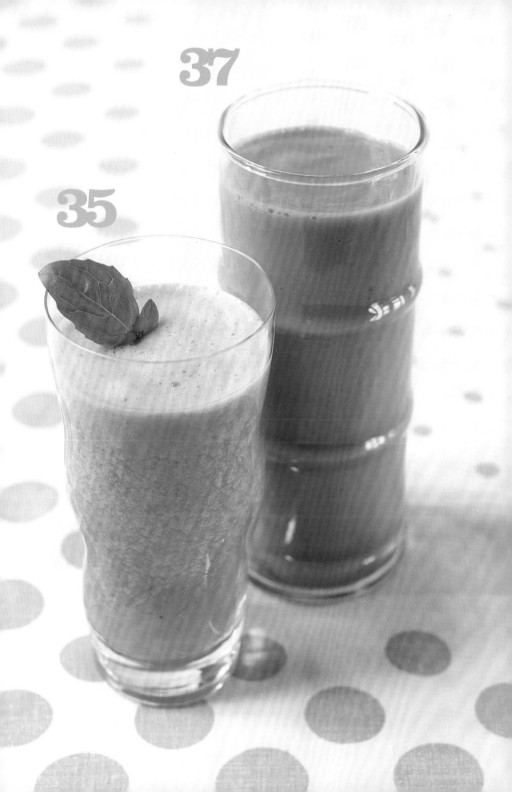

# 38

## peach + tofu smoothie

SERVES 2

100 g (3½ oz) peach
100 g (3½ oz) tofu
50 g (1¾ oz) vanilla ice cream
few drops of natural almond essence
100 ml (3½ fl oz) still mineral water
ice cubes

Peel, halve and stone the peach, then roughly chop the flesh.

Put the peach in a blender or smoothie maker, add the tofu, ice cream, almond essence and measured water and blend until smooth.

Pour the smoothie over ice cubes in glasses and serve immediately.

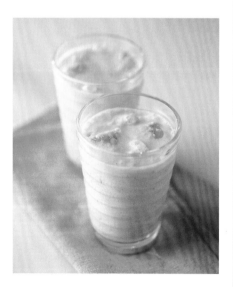

# 39

## cranberry, lemon + banana smoothie

SERVES 1

1 large banana
40 g (1½ oz) dried cranberries
juice of ½ lemon
1 tablespoon sesame seeds
2 tablespoons Greek yogurt
200 ml (7 fl oz) milk
crushed ice

Peel the banana, then roughly chop.

Put the dried cranberries and lemon juice in a blender or smoothie maker and blend until the berries are finely chopped.

Add the banana and sesame seeds and blend together.

Finally, add the yogurt and milk and blend until smooth and frothy.

Pour the smoothie over crushed ice in a glass and serve immediately.

This smoothie is rich in calcium (vital for bones and cell repair) and also has useful amounts of iron (good for blood) and zinc, which is essential for healing body tissue.

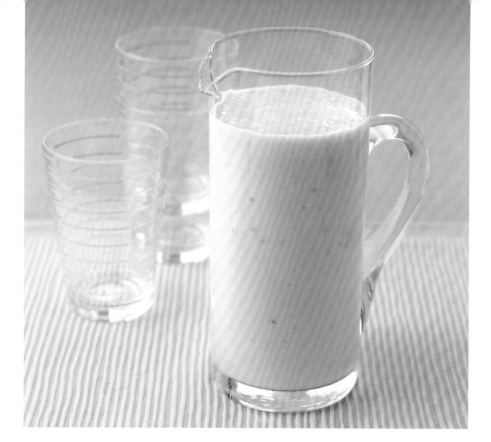

# 40

## apple, banana + wheatgerm
### smoothie

SERVES 3–4

2 tablespoons wheatgerm

1 tablespoon sesame seeds

2 bananas

75 g (2¾ oz) pineapple

450 ml (16 fl oz) fresh apple juice

300 g (10½ oz) live natural yogurt

Spread the wheatgerm and sesame seeds over a baking sheet and toast gently under a preheated medium grill until the sesame seeds have begun to turn golden brown, stirring a couple of times. Remove from the grill and leave to cool.

Peel and slice the bananas. Cut the skin off the pineapple and remove the core, then roughly chop the flesh.

Put the bananas and pineapple in a blender or smoothie maker and blend to a coarse purée. Add the apple juice and blend again to make a smooth juice. Finally, add the yogurt and the cooled wheatgerm and sesame seeds and blend again.

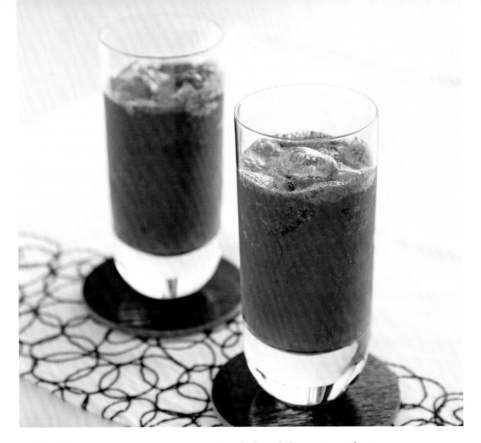

# 41

## oaty blackberry, date + almond milk smoothie

SERVES 2

1 beetroot

6 semi-dried dates

1 tablespoon rolled oats

100 g (3½ oz) blackberries

1 teaspoon maca powder

500 ml (18 fl oz) almond milk

1 teaspoon ground flax seeds

ice cubes

Trim the beetroot and then scrub or peel. Stone the dates.

Juice the beetroot.

Transfer the beetroot juice to a blender or smoothie maker, add all the remaining ingredients except the ice cubes and blend until smooth.

Pour the smoothie over ice cubes in glasses and serve immediately.

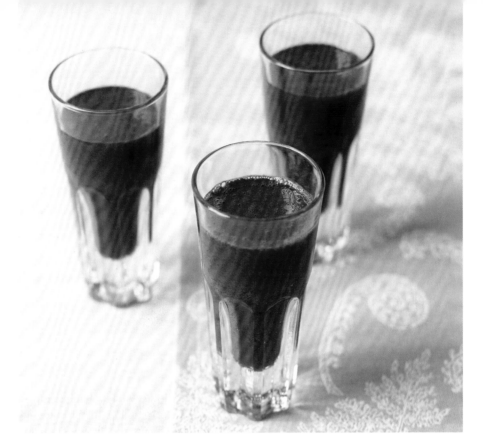

# 42

## spiced blackberry + kale
### smoothie

SERVES 1

2 apples

25 g (1 oz) kale

½ lemon

150 g (5½ oz) blackberries

100 g (3½ oz) natural yogurt

1 teaspoon ground flax seeds

¼ –½ teaspoon ground
   cinnamon

Remove the stalks from the apples. Cut any really
woody stalks off the kale. Peel the lemon.

Juice the kale, lemon and apples together.

Transfer the juice to a blender or smoothie maker,
add all the remaining ingredients and blend until
smooth.

Pour the smoothie into a glass and serve
immediately.

# 43

## broccoli, spinach + tomato juice

SERVES 1

**150 g (5½ oz) broccoli**

**150 g (5½ oz) spinach**

**2 tomatoes**

**celery stick, to decorate (optional)**

Trim the broccoli and rinse the spinach.

Juice the green vegetables with the tomatoes, adding the broccoli and spinach alternately so that the spinach leaves do not clog the juicer.

Pour the juice into a glass, add a stick of celery, if liked, and serve immediately.

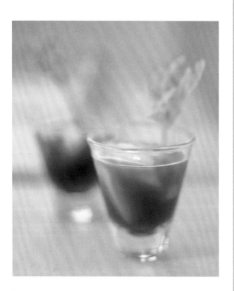

# 44

## gingery fig, strawberry + beetroot smoothie

SERVES 2

**1 beetroot**

**100 g (3½ oz) strawberries**

**3-cm (1¼-inch) piece fresh root ginger**

**6 figs**

**1 lemon grass stalk**

**1 tablespoon rolled oats**

**1 teaspoon maca powder**

**500 ml (18 fl oz) almond milk**

Trim the beetroot and then scrub or peel. Hull the strawberries. Peel the ginger. Remove the stalks from the figs, then roughly chop.

Juice the beetroot, ginger and lemon grass stalk together.

Transfer the juice to a blender or smoothie maker, add the remaining ingredients and blend until smooth.

Pour the smoothie into glasses and serve immediately.

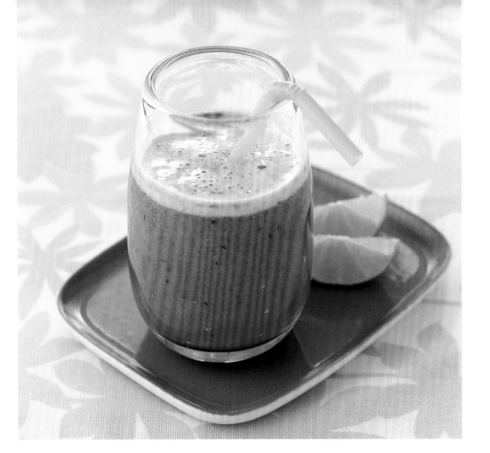

# 45

## tomato, red pepper + cabbage juice

SERVES 1

**175 g (6 oz) red pepper**
**100 g (3½ oz) white cabbage**
**175 g (6 oz) tomatoes**
**1 tablespoon chopped parsley**
**lime wedge, to decorate (optional)**

Core and deseed the red pepper. Trim the cabbage.

Juice the pepper, cabbage and tomatoes together.

Pour the juice into a glass and stir in the parsley, then decorate with a lime wedge, if liked, and serve immediately.

# 46

## next time...

Trim 4 celery sticks and cut them into 5-cm (2-inch) lengths. Juice the celery with 3 ripe tomatoes and half a red pepper. Add a crushed garlic clove and chopped chilli, to taste.

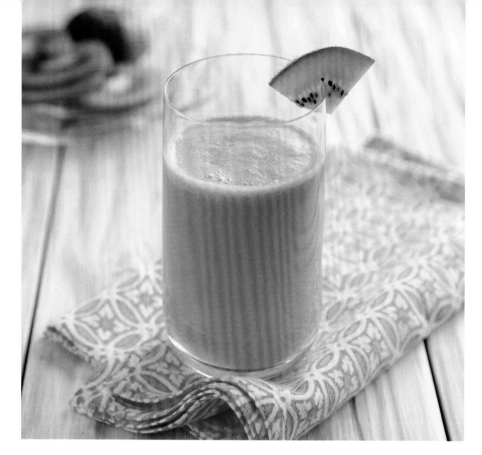

# 47

## apricot, pineapple + carrot juice

SERVES 1

**1 orange**

**1 kiwifruit, plus an extra slice to decorate**

**2 apricots**

**180 g (6¼ oz) pineapple**

**1 large carrot**

Peel the orange and kiwifruit. Halve and stone the apricots. Cut the skin off the pineapple and remove the core if very tough. Take the top off the carrot and then scrub.

Juice all the ingredients together.

Pour the juice into a glass, decorate with a kiwifruit slice and serve immediately.

# 48

**next time...**

Fancy some bubbles? Top up this juice with some sparkling mineral water to make a refreshing long drink.

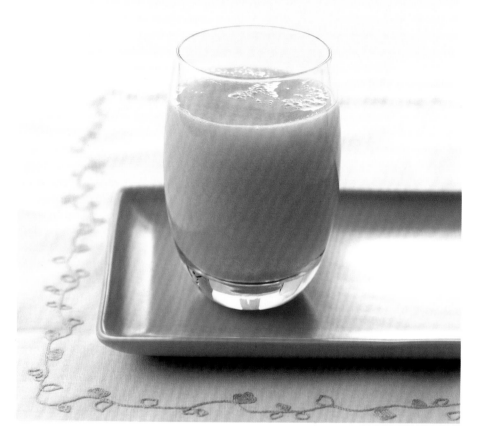

# 49

## pineapple, grape + celery
juice

SERVES 1

**125 g (4½ oz) pineapple**

**50 g (1¾ oz) celery**

**125 g (4½ oz) green seedless
grapes**

**50 g (1¾ oz) lettuce, plus
extra leaves to decorate
(optional)**

**2–3 ice cubes (optional)**

Cut the skin off the pineapple and remove the core
if very tough, then roughly chop the flesh. Peel
away any stringy bits from the celery. Separate the
lettuce leaves.

Juice the pineapple and celery with the grapes and
lettuce.

Pour the juice over ice cubes, if using, in a glass,
decorate with extra lettuce leaves, if liked, and
serve immediately.

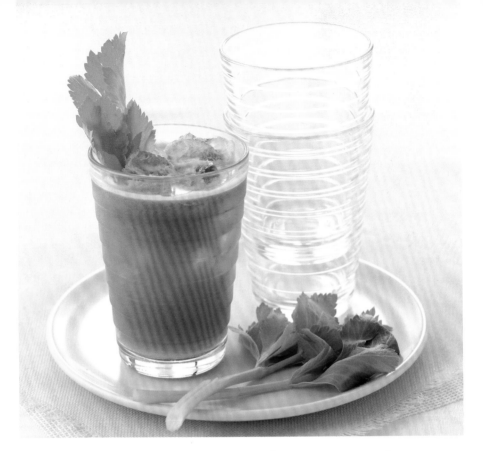

# 50

## tomato, lemon + parsley
juice

SERVES 1

**2 celery sticks, plus extra leaves to decorate**

**4 tomatoes**

**large handful of parsley**

**grated zest and juice of ½ lemon**

**ice cubes**

Peel away any stringy bits from the celery.

Juice the celery with the tomatoes, parsley and lemon zest and juice.

Pour the juice over ice cubes in a glass, decorate with celery leaves, if liked, and serve immediately.

# 51

## next time...

Replace the lemon juice and rind and the parsley with Tabasco, celery salt and black pepper.

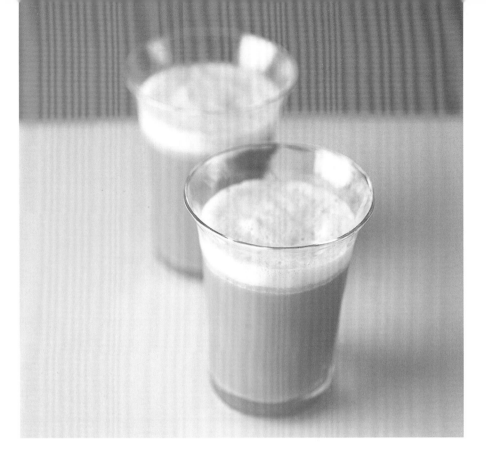

# 52

## celery, ginger + pineapple
juice

SERVES 1

**125 g (4½ oz) celery**

**125 g (4½ oz) pineapple**

**2.5-cm (1-inch) piece fresh
root ginger**

**crushed ice**

Peel away any stringy bits from the celery. Cut the skin off the pineapple and remove the core if very tough, then roughly chop the flesh. Peel the ginger.

Juice all the prepared ingredients together. Transfer the juice to a blender or food processor and blend with a little crushed ice.

Pour the juice into a glass and serve immediately.

# 53

## next time...

Juice 100 g (3½ oz) each of celery, any stringy bits removed, and fennel, trimmed, with ½ grapefruit, peeled. Serve over crushed ice.

**41**

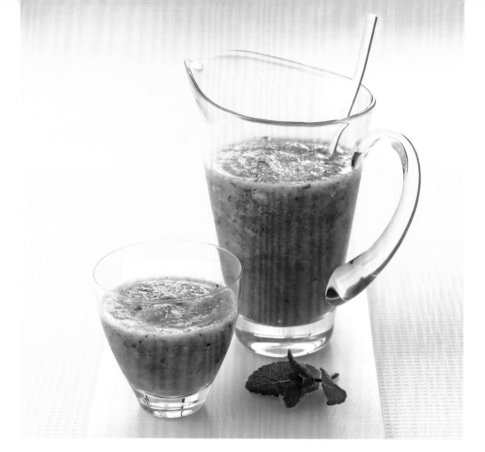

# 54

## watermelon + strawberry
juice

SERVES 1

**200 g (7 oz) strawberries**

**200 g (7 oz) watermelon**

**small handful of mint
leaves, plus extra sprigs
to decorate (optional)**

**2–3 ice cubes**

Hull the strawberries. Peel the watermelon as close to the skin as possible and deseed, then roughly chop the flesh.

Put the fruits in a blender or food processor, add the mint and ice cubes and blend briefly.

Pour the juice into a glass, decorate with mint sprigs, if liked, and serve immediately.

# 55

## pomelo + grapefruit
smoothie

SERVES 1

**1 pomelo**
**1 red grapefruit**
**100 ml (3½ fl oz) soya milk**
**2-3 teaspoons clear honey**
**ice cubes**

Peel the pomelo and grapefruit and then juice the fruits.

Transfer the juice to a bowl, add the soya milk and honey and whisk with an electric whisk until a thick froth forms on the surface.

Pour the smoothie over ice cubes in a glass and serve immediately.

# 56

## pear + pineapple juice

SERVES 1

**200 g (7 oz) fresh or canned pineapple**
**½ lemon**
**2 pears**
**ice cubes**

If using fresh pineapple, cut off the skin and remove the core, then roughly chop the flesh. If using canned pineapple, drain and discard the juice. Juice the lemon with the pineapple and pears.

Pour the juice into a glass over ice cubes and serve immediately.

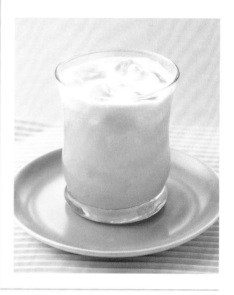

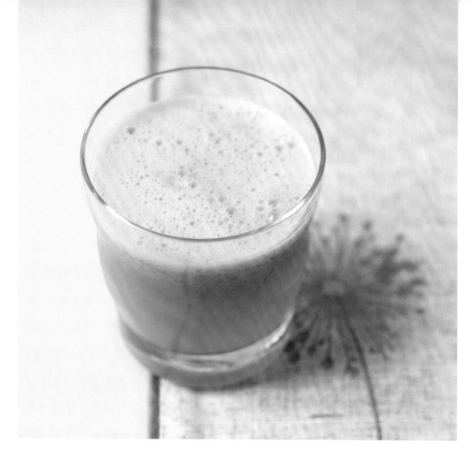

# 57

## grapefruit, fennel + spinach
juice

SERVES 1

**2 grapefruits**

**20 g (¾ oz) spinach**

**25 g (1 oz) fennel**

**100 ml (3½ fl oz) coconut water**

**½–1 teaspoon agave syrup**

Peel the grapefruits and rinse the spinach.

Juice the grapefruits, spinach and fennel together.

Transfer to a blender or food processor, add the coconut water and agave syrup and blend briefly.

Pour the juice into a glass and serve immediately.

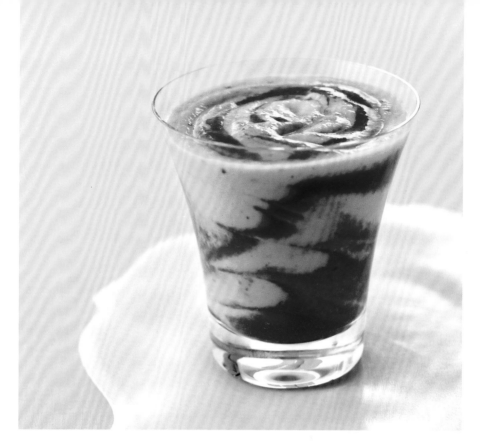

# 58

## marbled peach
milkshake

SERVES 2

**300 g (10½ oz) raspberries**

**4 teaspoons clear honey**

**2 large peaches**

**1 teaspoon vanilla bean paste
or a few drops of vanilla
extract**

**125 ml (4 fl oz) single cream**

**150 ml (5 fl oz) fresh orange
juice**

Put the raspberries in a blender or smoothie maker and blend to a purée. Press through a non-metallic strainer to remove the seeds and stir in half the honey. Check the sweetness, adding a little more honey if necessary.

Halve and stone the peaches, then roughly chop the flesh. Blend the peaches with the vanilla bean paste or extract and cream until smooth. Blend in the orange juice and any remaining honey.

Spoon a layer of the peach purée to a depth of about 2 cm (¾ inch) into glasses. Add a layer of raspberry purée and repeat the layering. Lightly marble the layers together with a knife and serve immediately.

# 59

## carrot + Brazil nut juice

SERVES 1

2 carrots

1 apple

2-cm (¾-inch) piece fresh root ginger

3 Brazil nuts

Take the tops off the carrots and then scrub. Remove the stalk from the apple and peel the ginger.

Juice the carrots, then the nuts, ginger and apple in that order.

Pour the juice into a glass and serve immediately.

# 60

## kefir + berry smoothie

SERVES 1

1 orange

200 g (7 oz) kefir

150 g (5½ oz) frozen mixed summer berries

Peel and then juice the orange.

Transfer the juice to a blender or smoothie maker, add the kefir and berries and blend until smooth. Serve immediately.

# 61

## apple + oat smoothie

SERVES 1

1 apple

1 banana

150 g (5½ oz) live natural yogurt

200 ml (7 fl oz) skimmed milk

few drops of vanilla extract

2 teaspoons clear honey

2 tablespoons muesli

Remove the stalk from the apple, then roughly chop. Peel the banana, then roughly chop.

Put all the ingredients in a blender or smoothie maker and blend until smooth.

Pour the smoothie into a glass and serve immediately.

Add a handful of sunflower seeds to rev up the omega-3 levels.

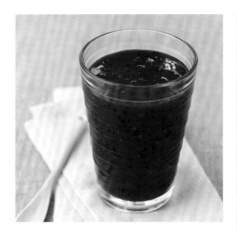

## 62

# beetroot + berry
## smoothie

SERVES 1

**50 g (1¾ oz) beetroot**

**100 g (3½ oz) blueberries, plus extra to decorate (optional)**

**100 g (3½ oz) raspberries**

**2–3 ice cubes**

Scrub or peel the beetroot and then juice.

Pour the beetroot juice into a blender or smoothie maker, add the blueberries, raspberries and ice cubes and blend until smooth.

Pour the smoothie into a glass, decorate with extra blueberries, if liked, and serve immediately.

## 63

# peach + pomegranate
## juice

SERVES 1

**2 peaches**

**1 apple**

**1 carrot**

**1 pomegranate**

Halve and stone the peaches. Remove the stalk from the apple. Take the top off the carrot and then scrub.

Remove the seeds from the pomegranate by cutting the fruit in half, then holding the halved fruit over a bowl and hitting the skin with a wooden spoon so that the seeds fall into the bowl.

Juice all the ingredients together.

Pour the juice into a glass and serve immediately.

## 64
### next time...

Juice 2 peaches with 3 pears for a thick, nutritious drink.

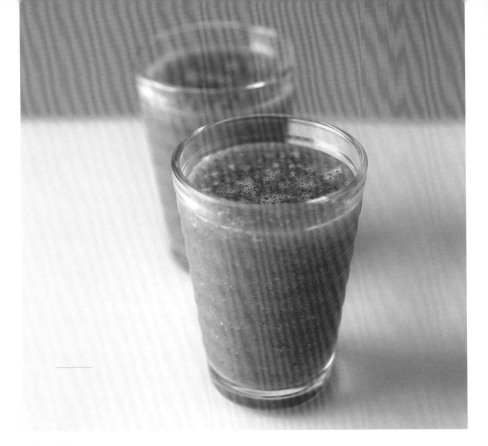

# 65

## watermelon cooler

SERVES 2

**100 g (3½ oz) watermelon**

**100 g (3½ oz) strawberries**

**100 ml (3½ fl oz) still mineral water**

**small handful of tarragon leaves**

Peel the watermelon as close to the skin as possible and deseed, then roughly chop the flesh. Hull the strawberries.

Put the watermelon and strawberries in a freezerproof container and freeze for 2 hours or overnight.

Transfer the frozen watermelon and strawberries to a blender or food processor, add the measured water and the tarragon and blend until smooth.

Pour the mixture into glasses and serve immediately.

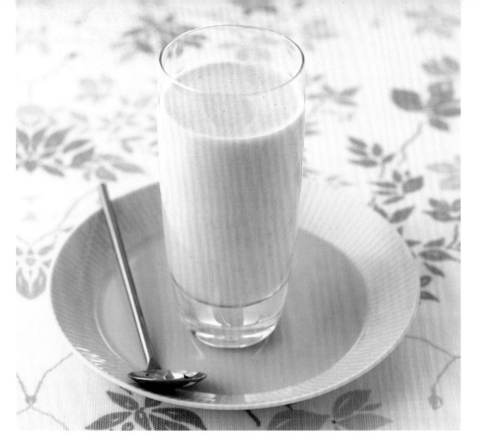

# 66

## banana + tahini smoothie

**SERVES 1**

**1 banana**

**300 ml (10 fl oz) semi-skimmed milk**

**2 teaspoons tahini paste**

Peel and slice the banana, put it in a freezerproof container and freeze for at least 2 hours or overnight.

Transfer the frozen banana to a blender or smoothie maker, add the milk and tahini paste and blend until smooth.

Pour the smoothie into a glass and serve immediately.

# 67
## next time...

Place 1 banana, 150 ml (5 fl oz) fresh orange juice and 25 g (1 oz) sunflower seeds in a blender or smoothie maker and blend together.

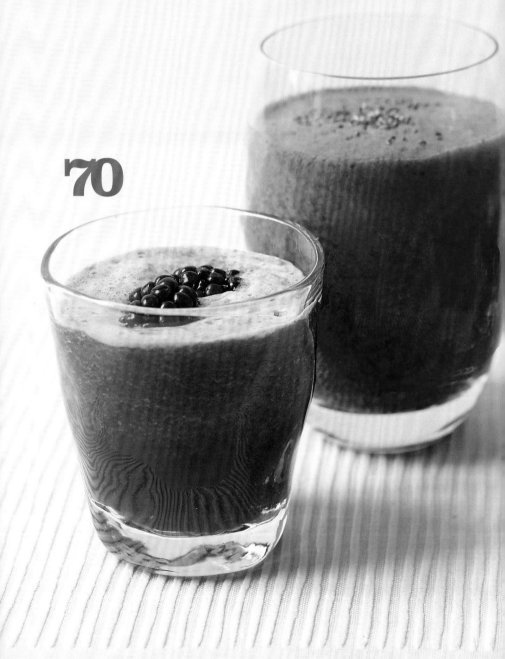

69

70

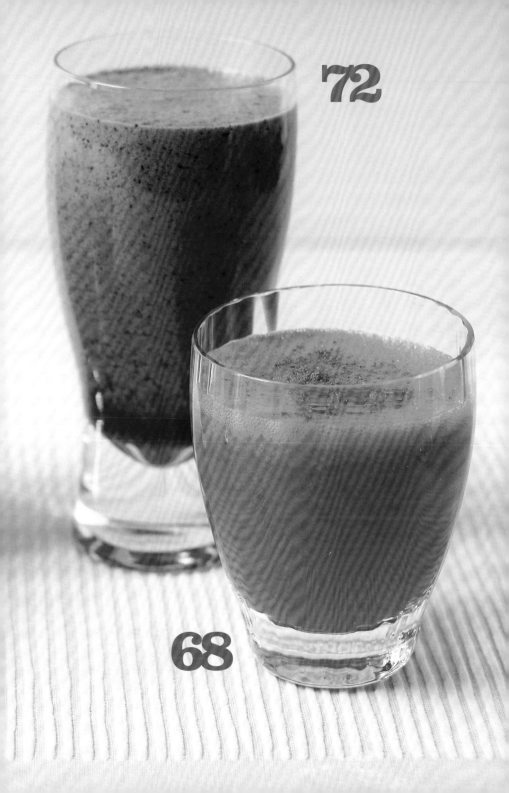

72

68

# 69

## berry + chia smoothie

SERVES 1

75 g (2¾ oz) frozen mixed berries

125 ml (4 fl oz) pure pomegranate juice

75 ml (2½ fl oz) water

½ tablespoon chia seeds, plus extra to
decorate

Put all ingredients in a blender or
smoothie maker and blend until
smooth.

Pour the smoothie into a glass,
sprinkle some chia seeds on top and
serve immediately.

# 68

## strawberry + red pepper juice

SERVES 1

200 g (7 oz) strawberries

1 apple

½ red pepper

1 teaspoon freshly squeezed lime juice

pinch of chilli powder, to taste, plus
extra to decorate

Hull the strawberries. Remove the
stalk from the apple. Core and deseed
the red pepper.

Juice the strawberries, apple and red
pepper together, then stir in the lime
juice and add chilli powder to taste.
Pour the juice into a glass, sprinkle
some chilli powder on top and serve
immediately.

# 70

## blackberry, apple + cucumber juice

SERVES 1

1 sweet apple

½ cucumber

200 g (7 oz) blackberries, plus one
blackberry, halved, to decorate

Remove the stalk from the apple. Trim
the cucumber.

Juice the apple, then the cucumber and
blackberries.

Pour the juice into a glass, decorate
with the blackberry halves and serve
immediately.

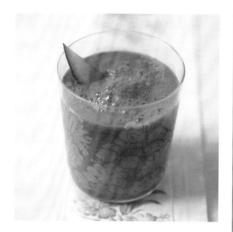

## 72

# blueberry + walnut
## smoothie

SERVES 1

**125 ml (4 fl oz) pure pomegranate juice**
**100 g (3½ oz) blueberries**
**75 g (2¾ oz) low-fat Greek yogurt**
**10 g (¼ oz) walnuts**

Put all the ingredients in a blender or smoothie maker and blend until smooth.

Pour the smoothie into a glass and serve immediately.

## 71

# watermelon +
# clementine juice

SERVES 1

**200 g (7 oz) watermelon, plus a thin slice to decorate**
**3–4 clementines**

Peel the watermelon as close to the skin as possible and deseed, then roughly chop the flesh. Peel the clementines.

Juice the fruits together.

Pour the juice into a glass, top with the watermelon slice and serve immediately.

## 73

# carrot + stinging nettle
## juice

SERVES 1

**2 carrots**
**1 lemon**
**1 apple**
**handful of stinging nettles**

Take the tops off the carrots and then scrub. Peel the lemon. Remove the stalk from the apple.

Juice all the ingredients together.

Pour the juice into a glass and serve immediately

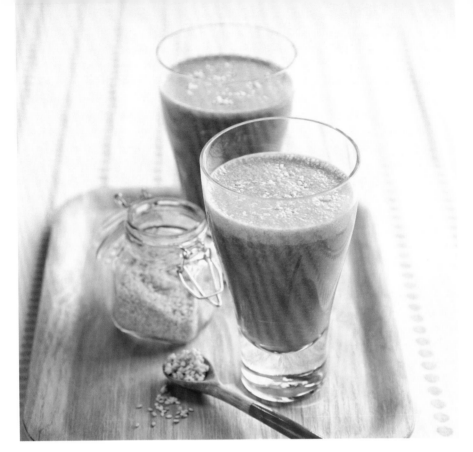

## 74

### beetroot, kale + hemp milk
smoothie

SERVES 2

**1 beetroot**

**50 g (1¾ oz) strawberries**

**25 g (1 oz) kale**

**1 banana**

**25 g (1 oz) cranberries**

**50 g (1¾ oz) pomegranate seeds**

**1 tablespoon goji berries**

**500 ml (18 fl oz) hemp milk**

**1 tablespoon avocado oil**

**1 tablespoon toasted sesame seeds, to decorate**

Trim the beetroot and then scrub or peel. Hull the strawberries. Cut any really tough stalks off the kale. Peel the banana, then roughly chop.

Juice the beetroot, kale, cranberries and pomegranate seeds together.

Transfer the juice to a blender or smoothie maker, add all the remaining ingredients except the toasted sesame seeds and blend until smooth.

Pour the smoothie into glasses, sprinkle with the toasted sesame seeds and serve immediately.

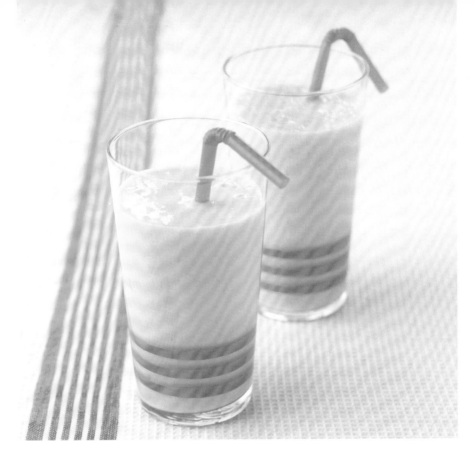

# 75

## banana, orange + mango
smoothie

SERVES 2

**1 banana**

**1 mango**

**200 ml (7 fl oz) fresh orange juice**

**200 ml (7 fl oz) skimmed milk**

**3 tablespoons fromage frais**

Peel the banana, then roughly chop. Peel and stone the mango, then roughly chop the flesh.

Put the banana and mango in a blender or smoothie maker, add the orange juice, milk and fromage frais and blend until smooth.

Pour the smoothie into glasses and serve immediately.

# 76

## next time...

Blend 1 small banana, peeled and roughly chopped, and 1 small avocado, peeled and stoned, with 250 ml (9 fl oz) skimmed milk until smooth.

**55**

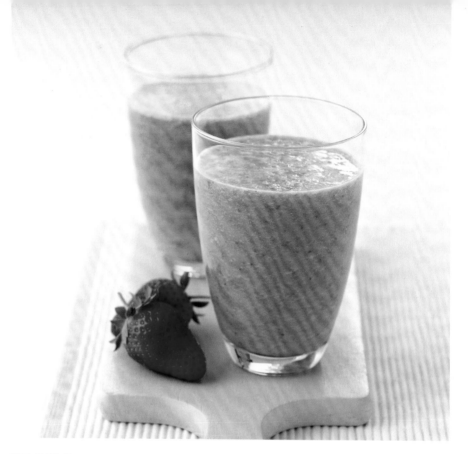

 **77**

### orange, mango + strawberry
smoothie

SERVES 1

**125 g (4½ oz) strawberries,
plus extra to decorate
(optional)**

**1 small mango**

**300 ml (10 fl oz) fresh orange
juice**

Hull the strawberries, then put them in a
freezerproof container and freeze for 2 hours
or overnight.

Peel and stone the mango, then roughly chop the
flesh. Put in a blender or smoothie maker with the
frozen strawberries and orange juice and blend
until smooth.

Pour the smoothie into a glass, decorate with extra
strawberries, if liked, and serve immediately.

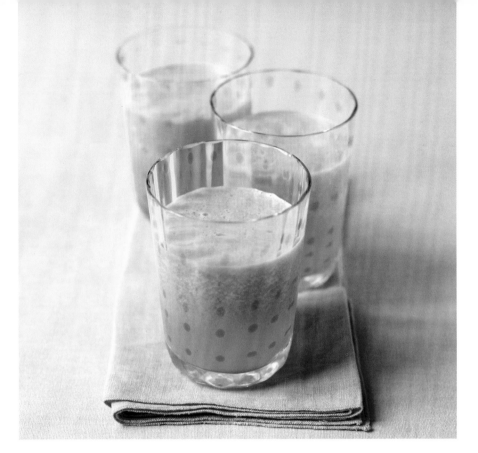

78

## cucumber, pineapple
## + mint juice

SERVES 1

**½ pineapple**

**½ small cucumber**

**8 mint leaves, plus extra to
decorate (optional)**

Cut the skin off the pineapple and remove the core
if very tough, then roughly chop the flesh. Trim the
cucumber.

Juice all the ingredients together.

Pour the juice into a glass, decorate with extra
mint leaves, if liked, and serve immediately.

## 79

## apple, orange + berry
## smoothie

SERVES 1

**2 oranges**
**1 apple**
**150 g (5½ oz) strawberries**
**150 g (5½ oz) raspberries**
**150 g (5½ oz) live natural yogurt**

Peel the oranges and remove the stalk from the apple. Hull the strawberries.

Juice the oranges and apple together.

Transfer the juice to a blender or smoothie maker, add the berries and yogurt and blend until smooth.

Pour the smoothie into a glass and serve immediately.

**tip**

The combination of the pectin in the apple and probiotics in the yogurt makes this smoothie a great choice for the digestive tract.

## 80

## black tea, mango
## + spice smoothie

SERVES 1

**1 mango**
**2-cm (¾-inch) piece fresh root ginger**
**125 ml (4 fl oz) black tea, chilled**
**pinch of ground cinnamon**

Peel and stone the mango, then roughly chop the flesh. Peel the ginger.

Put the mango and ginger in a blender or smoothie maker, add the remaining ingredients and blend until smooth.

Pour the smoothie into a glass and serve immediately.

## 81

## lychee + pineapple juice

SERVES 1

**10 fresh lychees**
**½ pineapple**
**½ lime**

Peel and stone the lychees. Cut the skin off the pineapple and remove the core if very tough, then roughly chop the flesh.

Juice the lychees and pineapple with the unpeeled lime half.

Pour the juice into a glass and serve immediately.

## 82

## tomato, red pepper + papaya juice

SERVES 1

**125 g (4½ oz) papaya**
**100 g (3½ oz) red pepper**
**1 large tomato**
**2–3 ice cubes**

Peel and deseed the papaya. Core and deseed the red pepper.

Juice the papaya and red pepper with the tomato.

Transfer the juice to a blender or food processor, add the ice cubes and blend briefly.

Pour the juice into a glass and serve immediately.

## 83

## broccoli, carrot + beetroot juice

SERVES 1

**250 g (9 oz) broccoli**
**175 g (6 oz) carrots**
**50 g (1¾ oz) beetroot**

Trim the broccoli. Take the tops off the carrots and then scrub. Scrub or peel the beetroot.

Juice all the ingredients together.

Pour the juice into a glass and serve immediately.

## 84

## Earl grey + berry smoothie

SERVES 1

**125 ml (4 fl oz) Earl Grey tea, chilled**
**75 g (2¾ oz) frozen blueberries**
**75 g (2¾ oz) blackberries**

Put all the ingredients in a blender or smoothie maker and blend until smooth.

Pour the smoothie into a glass and serve immediately.

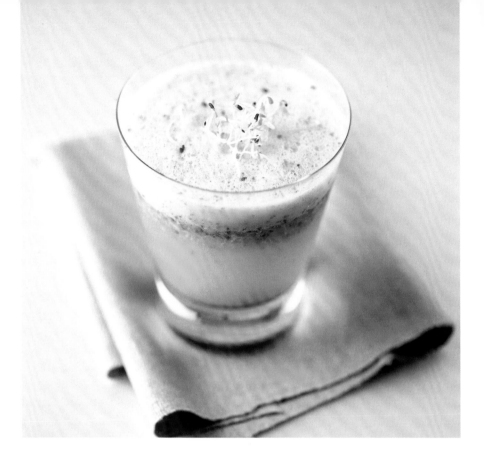

# 85

## pineapple + alfalfa
juice

SERVES 1

**150 g (5½ oz) pineapple**

**150 g (5½ oz) alfalfa sprouts,
plus extra to decorate**

**2–3 ice cubes**

**50 ml (2 fl oz) still mineral
water**

Cut the skin off the pineapple and remove the
core if very tough, then roughly chop the flesh.
Rinse the alfalfa sprouts.

Juice the pineapple.

Transfer the juice to a blender or food processor,
add the alfalfa sprouts, ice cubes and measured
water and blend briefly.

Pour the juice into a glass, decorate with extra
alfalfa sprouts and serve immediately.

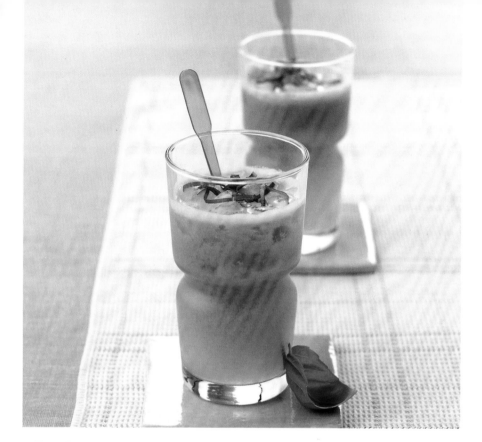

# 86

## tomato, apple + basil
juice

SERVES 1

**1 celery stick**

**1 apple**

**4 large tomatoes**

**ice cubes**

**4 basil leaves, finely chopped,
plus extra, shredded, to
decorate**

**1½ tablespoons freshly
squeezed lime juice**

Peel away any stringy bits from the celery.
Remove the stalk from the apple.

Juice the celery, apple and tomatoes together.

Pour the juice over ice cubes in a glass and stir
in the chopped basil and lime juice. Add extra
shredded basil leaves and serve immediately.

## pineapple, broccoli + kiwifruit juice

SERVES 1

**200 g (7 oz) pineapple**
**100 g (3½ oz) broccoli**
**100 g (3½ oz) cucumber**
**1 kiwifruit**
**2 ice cubes**

Cut the skin off the pineapple and remove the core if very tough, then roughly chop the flesh. Trim the broccoli and the cucumber. Peel the kiwifruit.

Juice the pineapple and broccoli together.

Transfer the juice to a blender or food processor, add the cucumber, kiwifruit and the ice cubes and blend until smooth.

Pour the juice into a glass and serve immediately.

## grapefruit + cucumber fizz

SERVES 1

**300 g (10½ oz) grapefruit**
**½ lemon**
**350 g (12 oz) cucumber**
**sparkling mineral water, for topping up**
**a few mint leaves, chopped**

Peel the grapefruit and lemon. Trim the cucumber.

Juice the prepared ingredients together.

Pour the juice into a glass, then top up with sparkling mineral water, stir in the chopped mint and serve immediately.

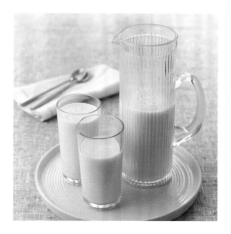

## 90

### spiced melon juice

SERVES 1

**250 g (9 oz) cantaloupe melon**
**500 g (1 lb 2oz) watermelon**
**50 g (1¾ oz) spinach**
**2-cm (¾-inch) piece fresh root ginger**
**2-3 ice cubes**
**grated nutmeg, to decorate**

Peel both melons as close to the skin as possible and deseed, then roughly chop the flesh. Rinse the spinach. Peel the ginger.

Juice the prepared ingredients together.

Transfer the juice to a blender or food processor, add the ice cubes and blend briefly.

Pour into a glass, sprinkle with nutmeg to decorate and serve immediately.

## 89

### mango, coconut + lime lassi

SERVES 2

**1 large mango**
**juice of 1 orange**
**juice of 1 lime**
**1 tablespoon clear honey**
**300 g (10½ oz) natural yogurt**
**4 tablespoons coconut milk**
**ice cubes**

Peel and stone the mango, then roughly chop the flesh.

Put the mango in a blender or smoothie maker, add the orange and lime juices, honey, yogurt and coconut milk and blend until smooth.

Pour over ice cubes in glasses and serve immediately.

## 91

### next time...

Replace the spinach with 1 large carrot, about 150 g (5½ oz), top trimmed and then scrubbed.

# 92

## carrot + lettuce juice

SERVES 1

**100 g (3½ oz) carrots**
**200 g (7 oz) lettuce**
**ice cubes**
**chopped coriander leaves, to decorate**

Take the tops off the carrots and then scrub. Separate the lettuce leaves.

Juice the carrot with the lettuce, taking care that the lettuce leaves do not clog the machine.

Pour the juice over ice cubes in a glass, decorate with chopped coriander and serve immediately.

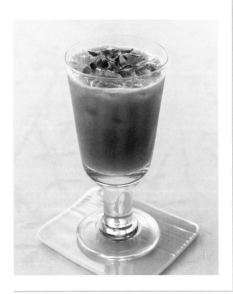

# 93

## mango, spinach + cashew smoothie

SERVES 1

**½ large mango**
**25 g (1 oz) spinach**
**75 ml (2½ fl oz) skimmed milk or almond milk**
**75 ml (2½ fl oz) freshly squeezed orange juice**
**1 heaped teaspoon cashew nut butter**
**juice of ½ lime**

Peel the mango, then roughly chop the flesh. Rinse the spinach.

Put the mango and spinach in a blender or smoothie maker, add all the other ingredients and blend until smooth.

Pour the smoothie into a glass and serve immediately.

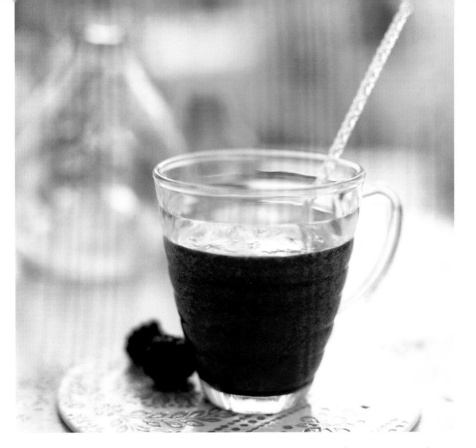

# 94

## blackberry, cantaloupe melon + kiwifruit juice

SERVES 1

**100 g (3½ oz) cantaloupe melon**

**2 kiwifruits**

**100 g (3½ oz) fresh or frozen blackberries, plus extra to decorate**

**2–3 ice cubes**

Peel the melon as close to the skin as possible and deseed, then roughly chop the flesh. Peel the kiwifruits.

Juice the melon, kiwifruits and blackberries together.

Transfer the juice to a blender or food processor, add the ice cubes and blend briefly.

Pour the juice into a glass, decorate with a few extra blackberries and serve immediately.

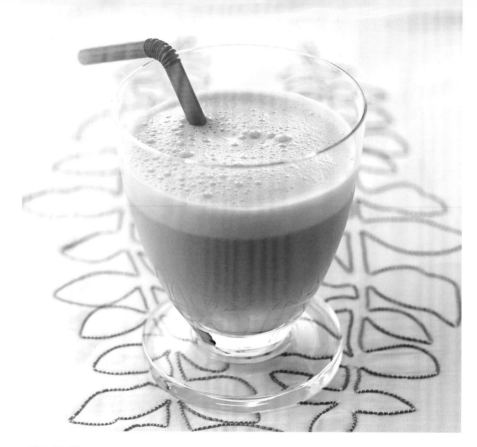

# 95

## cranberry + apple smoothie

SERVES 1

**250 g (9 oz) apples**

**100 g (3½ oz) frozen cranberries**

**100 g (3½ oz) live natural yogurt**

**1 tablespoon clear honey**

**ice cubes (optional)**

Remove the stalks from the apples and then juice.

Transfer the juice to a blender or smoothie maker, add the frozen cranberries, yogurt and honey and blend briefly.

Pour the smoothie over ice cubes, if using, in a glass and serve immediately.

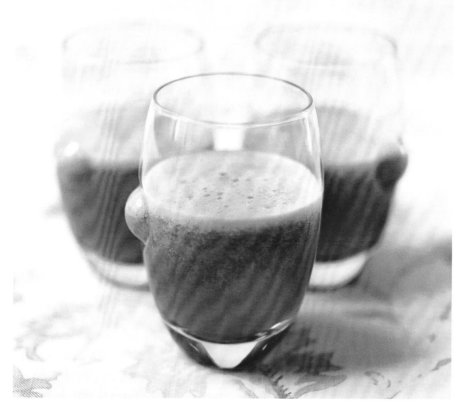

# 96

## apple, strawberry + celery
juice

SERVES 1

**2 celery sticks**

**150 g (5½ oz) strawberries**

**2 sweet apples**

Peel away any stringy bits from the celery. Hull the strawberries and remove the stalks from the apples.

Juice all the ingredients together.

Pour the juice into a glass and serve immediately.

# 97
next time...

Juice together 150 g (5½ oz) raspberries, 125 g (4½ oz) cucumber, trimmed, and 1 apple and 1 pear, stalks removed.

67

# 98

## minty summer vegetable juice

SERVES 1

½ cucumber

2 young carrots

small handful of mint, plus an extra sprig to decorate

6 asparagus spears

ice cubes

Trim the cucumber. Take the tops off the carrots and then scrub. Pull the mint leaves off their stalks.

Juice the prepared ingredients with the asparagus.

Pour the juice over ice cubes in a glass, decorate with a mint sprig and serve immediately.

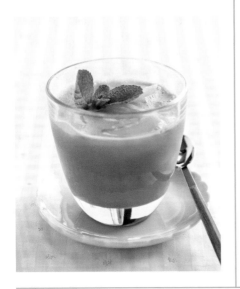

# 99

## clementine + stinging nettle infusion

SERVES 1

1 clementine

4 stinging nettle sprigs

200 ml (7 fl oz) boiling water

mild clear honey, to taste

Pare a long strip of rind from the clementine, then halve the clementine and squeeze the juice.

Put the clementine rind and stinging nettle sprigs in a cup, then pour over the measured boiling water and leave to infuse for 3–5 minutes.

Lift out the nettle sprigs and stir in the squeezed clementine juice and a little honey to taste. Serve immediately.

Like citrus fruits, nettles are rich in vitamin C and minerals, giving your system an invigorating boost.

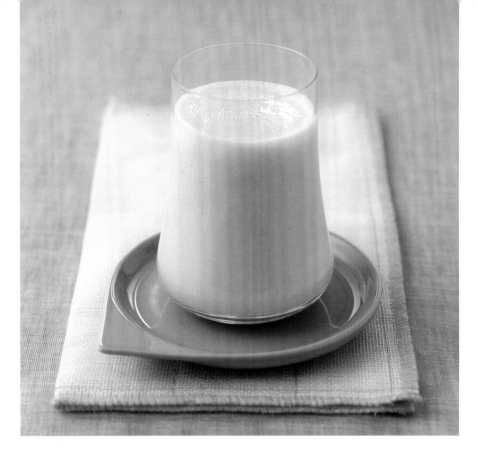

# 100

## creamy mango + pineapple
smoothie

SERVES 2

**1 large banana**

**1 large mango**

**150 g (5½ oz) natural yogurt**

**300 ml (10 fl oz) pineapple juice**

**pineapple chunks, to decorate (optional)**

Peel and slice the banana, then put it in a freezer-proof container and freeze for at least 2 hours or overnight.

Peel the mango, remove the stone and roughly chop the flesh. Place the flesh in a food processor or blender with the frozen banana, yogurt and pineapple juice and process until smooth.

Pour the mixture into glasses, decorate with pineapple chunks, if liked, and serve immediately.

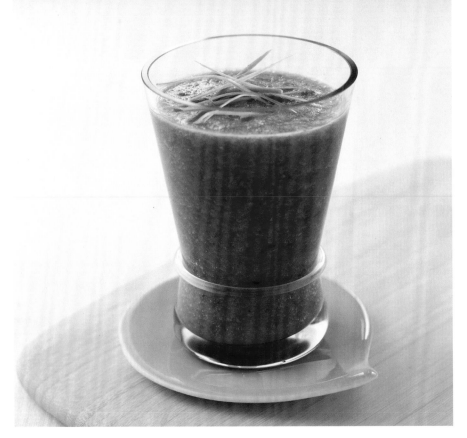

# 101

## red pepper + tomato
smoothie

SERVES 1

**50 g (1¾ oz) red pepper**

**50 g (1¾ oz) cucumber**

**30 g (1 oz) spring onion**

**100 ml (3½ fl oz) tomato juice**

**squeeze of lemon juice, to taste**

**splash of hot pepper sauce, to taste**

**splash of Worcestershire sauce, to taste**

**sea salt and freshly ground black pepper**

Core and deseed the red pepper, then roughly chop the flesh. Peel the cucumber, then roughly chop the flesh. Roughly chop the spring onion, reserving a few shreds to decorate.

Pour the tomato juice into a blender or smoothie maker, add the red pepper, cucumber and spring onion and blend briefly. Taste and then add lemon juice, hot pepper sauce, Worcestershire sauce and sea salt and black pepper to taste.

Pour the smoothie into a glass, decorate with the reserved spring onion shreds and serve immediately.

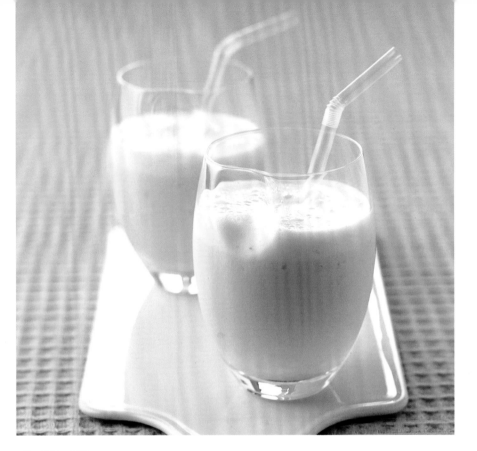

# 102

## cranberry + yogurt smoothie

SERVES 1

**100 g (3½ oz) cranberries**

**50 g (1¾ oz) Greek yogurt**

**100 ml (3½ fl oz) soya milk**

**2–3 ice cubes**

**1 teaspoon agave syrup (optional)**

Put the cranberries in a blender or smoothie maker, add the yogurt, soya milk and ice cubes and blend until smooth.

Stir in the agave syrup to sweeten, if liked, then blend again briefly.

Pour the smoothie into a glass and serve immediately.

# 103

## next time...

Blend 150 ml (5 fl oz) soya milk and 100 g (3½ oz) frozen raspberries together until smooth.

# 104

## passionfruit + banana
## smoothie

SERVES 2–3

**1 lime**

**2 bananas**

**4 passionfruits**

**600ml (20 fl oz) milk**

Peel and then juice the lime. Peel the bananas, then roughly chop.

Halve the passionfruits and scoop the seeds and pulp into a blender or smoothie maker. Add the lime juice, bananas and milk and blend until smooth.

Pour the smoothie into glasses and serve immediately.

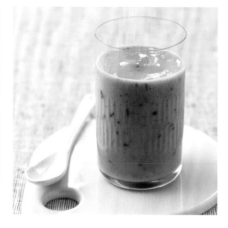

# 105

## dried fruit + apple
## smoothie

SERVES 2

**125 g (4½ oz) dried fruit salad**

**400 ml (14 fl oz) apple juice**

**200 ml (7 fl oz) Greek yogurt**

**ice cubes (optional)**

Roughly chop the dried fruit salad and place it in a large bowl. Pour over the apple juice, cover the bowl and leave to stand overnight.

Put the dried fruit salad and apple juice in a food processor or blender, add the yogurt and process until smooth, adding a little more apple juice if necessary.

Pour the smoothie into glasses, add a couple of ice cubes, if using, and serve immediately.

# 106

## raspberry + banana
## **yogurt** smoothie

SERVES 1

½ **banana**

**150 g (5½ oz) raspberries**

**100 g (3½ oz) natural yogurt**

**fresh apple juice, as needed**

Peel the banana. Put in a blender or smoothie maker with the raspberries, add the yogurt and blend until smooth.

Blend in as much apple juice as needed to achieve your desired consistency.

Pour the smoothie into a glass and serve immediately.

# 107

## next time...

Blend 125 g (4½ oz) strawberries, hulled, and 30 g (1 oz) redcurrants, stalks removed, with the yogurt, adding apple juice as required as above.

# 108

## gingery apple, mint
## **+ fennel** juice

SERVES 1

**2 apples**

**2-cm (¾-inch) piece fresh root ginger**

½ **fennel bulb**

**8 mint leaves**

Remove the stalks from the apples. Peel the ginger. Trim the fennel.

Juice all the ingredients together.

Pour the juice into a glass and serve immediately.

# 109

## mango, orange + cranberry juice

SERVES 1

**1 mango**
**1 orange**
**125 g (4½ oz) cranberries**
**100 ml (3½ fl oz) still mineral water**
**1 teaspoon clear honey**
**ice cubes (optional)**

Peel and stone the mango. Peel the orange.

Juice the orange with the mango and cranberries.

Pour the juice into a glass and stir in the measured water and honey. Add a couple of ice cubes, if using, and serve immediately.

# 110

## mango, apple + cucumber slush

SERVES 1

**200 g (7 oz) apple**
**125 g (4½ oz) cucumber**
**100 g (3½ oz) mango**
**ice cubes**

Peel the apple and cucumber. Peel the mango, remove the stone and roughly chop the flesh. Juice with the apples and cucumber.

Transfer the juice to a food processor or blender, add a couple of ice cubes and blend to make a fruity slush.

Serve immediately.

# 111

## next time...

Roughly chop the flesh of a peeled and stoned mango and add it to a food processor or blender with 150 ml (5 fl oz) live natural yogurt and the same amount of ice-cold still water, 1 tablespoon rosewater and ¼ teaspoon ground cardamom. Process briefly and serve immediately.

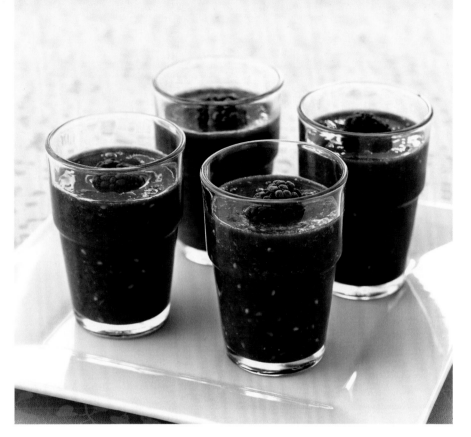

# 112

SERVES 1

**100 g (3½ oz) celeriac**

**50 g (1¾ oz) apple**

**100 g (3½ oz) frozen blackberries, plus extra to decorate**

**2–3 ice cubes**

## blackberry, apple + celeriac
juice

Peel the celeriac and cut into chunks. Juice the celeriac and apple together.

Transfer the juice to a blender or food processor, add the blackberries and ice cubes and blend briefly.

Pour the juice into a glass, decorate with extra blackberries and serve immediately.

# 113
## next time...

Juice 150 g (5½ oz) each of blackberries and pineapple with 25 g (1 oz) apple. Pour over ice cubes in a glass and serve immediately.

## 115

# chocolate + blackcurrant smoothie

SERVES 1

**¼ avocado**

**½ pear**

**30 g (1 oz) fresh or frozen (defrosted) blackcurrants with their stalks removed**

**100 ml (3½ fl oz) chocolate soya drink**

**1 square dark chocolate, grated, to decorate**

Peel the avocado and roughly chop the pear.

Put the avocado and pear in a blender or smoothie maker, add the blackcurrants and chocolate soya drink and blend until smooth.

Pour the smoothie into a glass, sprinkle with the chocolate and serve immediately.

## 114

# apple, banana + cinnamon shake

SERVES 1

**1 red apple**

**½ banana**

**3 raw almonds**

**100 g (3½ oz) Greek yogurt**

**100 ml (3½ fl oz) skimmed milk or almond milk**

**pinch of ground cinnamon, plus extra to decorate**

Remove the stalk from the apple. Peel the banana, then roughly chop.

Put the apple and banana in a blender or smoothie maker, add the almonds, yogurt, milk and cinnamon and blend until smooth.

Pour the shake into a glass, sprinkle some extra cinnamon on top and serve immediately.

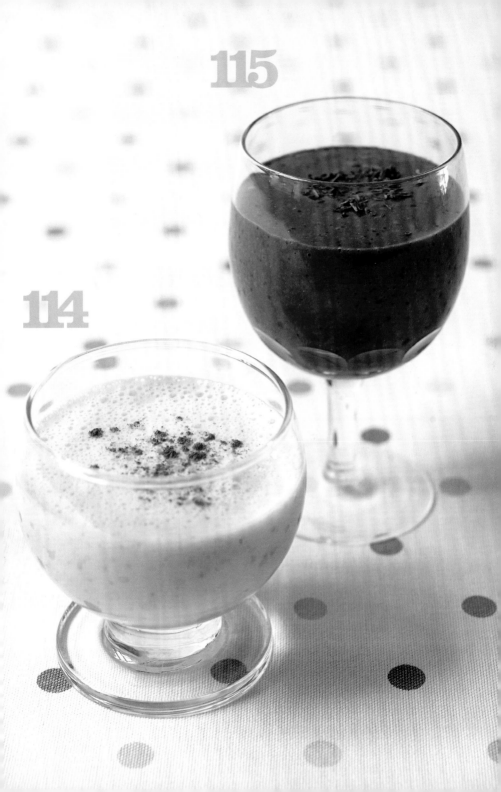

# 116

## summer berry + peach
### shake

SERVES 4

**2 peaches**
**300 g (10½ oz) strawberries**
**300 g (10½ oz) raspberries**
**400 ml (14 fl oz) milk**

Halve and stone the peaches, then roughly chop the flesh.

Put the peaches in a blender or smoothie maker with the strawberries and raspberries and blend until smooth.

Add the milk and blend again until the mixture is smooth and frothy.

Pour the shake into glasses and serve immediately.

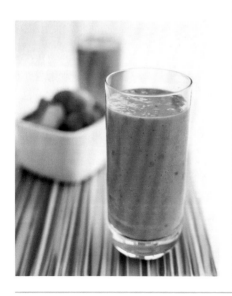

# 117

## tomato, cucumber
## + lemon juice

SERVES 1

**25 g (1 oz) cucumber, plus an extra slice to decorate**
**crushed ice**
**150 ml (5 fl oz) tomato juice**
**2 dashes of freshly squeezed lemon juice**
**2 dashes of Worcestershire sauce**
**sea salt and freshly ground black pepper**

Peel the cucumber.

Put a little crushed ice in a blender or food processor. Add the tomato juice, cucumber, lemon juice, Worcestershire sauce and sea salt and black pepper to taste and blend well.

Pour the juice into a glass, decorate with a cucumber slice on the rim and serve immediately.

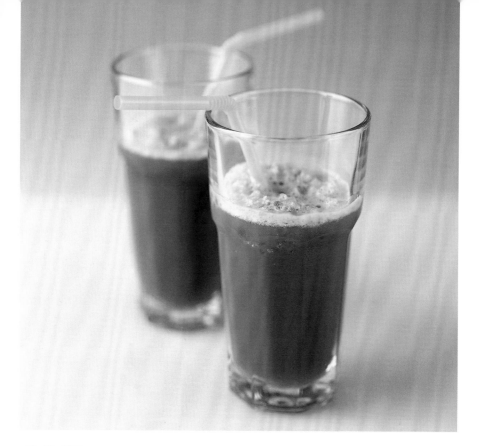

# 118

### celery + celeriac juice

SERVES 1

**150 g (5½ oz) celeriac**

**100 g (3½ oz) celery**

**100 g (3½ oz) lettuce**

**100 g (3½ oz) spinach**

**2-3 ice cubes**

Peel the celeriac and cut into chunks. Peel away any stringy bits from the celery. Separate the lettuce leaves. Rinse the spinach.

Juice all the prepared ingredients together, adding the lettuce and spinach alternately so that the leaves do not clog the machine.

Transfer the juice to a blender or food processor, add the ice cubes and blend briefly.

Pour the juice into a glass and serve immediately.

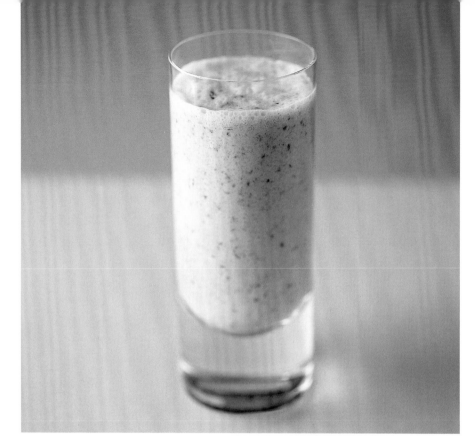

# 119

## **cucumber** lassi

SERVES 1

**150 g (5½ oz) cucumber**

**150 g (5½ oz) live natural yogurt**

**100 ml (3½ fl oz) ice-cold still mineral water**

**handful of mint**

**½ teaspoon ground cumin**

**squeeze of lemon juice**

Peel the cucumber, then roughly chop.

Put the cucumber in a blender or smoothie maker with the yogurt and measured water.

Pull the mint leaves off their stalks, reserving a few for decoration if liked. Chop the remainder roughly, add them to the blender or smoothie maker with the cumin and lemon juice and blend briefly.

Pour the lassi into a glass, decorate with the reserved mint leaves, if using, and serve immediately.

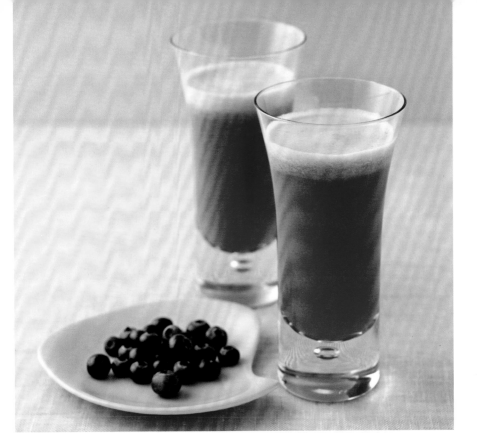

# 120

## blueberry, apple + ginger
juice

**SERVES 1**

**250 g (9 oz) apples**

**125 g (4½ oz) grapefruit**

**2.5-cm (1-inch) piece fresh
    root ginger**

**250 g (9 oz) blueberries**

**ice cubes (optional)**

Remove the stalks from the apples. Peel the grapefruit and ginger.

Juice the prepared ingredients with the blueberries.

Pour the juice over ice cubes, if using, in a glass, and serve immediately.

# 121

next time...

Juice 250 g (9 oz) apple with 2.5-cm (1-inch) piece fresh root ginger. If you like, top it up with ice-cold water.

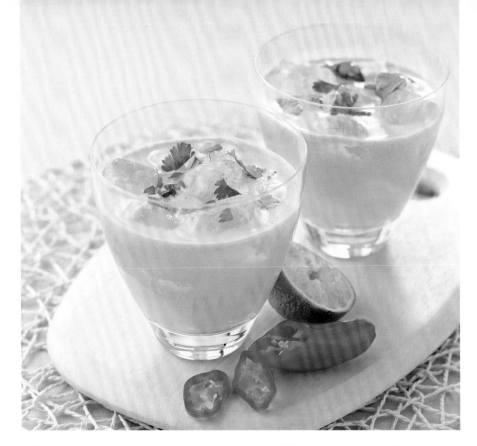

# 122

## carrot, chilli + pineapple
juice

**SERVES 1**

**250 g (9 oz) pineapple**

**250 g (9 oz) carrots**

**½ small chilli**

**ice cubes**

**juice of ½ lime**

**1 tablespoon chopped
coriander leaves**

Cut the skin off the pineapple and remove the core
if very tough, then roughly chop the flesh. Take
the tops off the carrots and then scrub. Deseed the
chilli.

Juice the pineapple, carrots and chilli together.

Pour the juice over ice cubes in a glass. Squeeze
over the lime juice, stir in the chopped coriander
and serve immediately.

**tip**

The chillies not only give this juice a bit of a kick,
they are also rich in carotenoids.

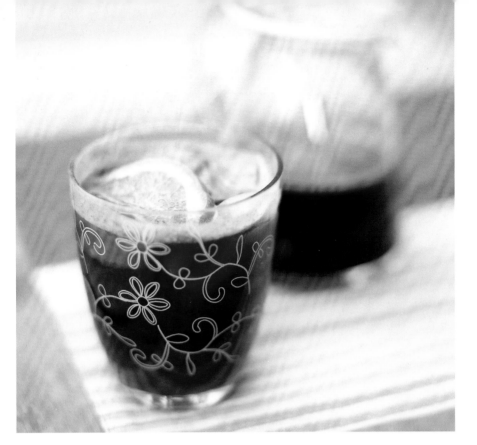

# 123

## carrot, cabbage + apple
juice

SERVES 1

**250 g (9 oz) apples**

**175 g (6 oz) carrots**

**125 g (4½ oz) red cabbage**

**ice cubes**

**orange slice, to decorate**

Remove the stalks from the apples. Take the tops off the carrots and then scrub. Trim the cabbage.

Juice the apples, carrots and cabbage together.

Pour the juice over ice cubes in a glass, decorate with an orange slice and serve immediately.

## 124

### apple, pear + spinach
lemonade

SERVES 1

**1 apple**

**1 pear**

**½ lemon**

**25 g (1 oz) spinach**

**¼ cucumber**

Remove the stalks from the apple and pear. Peel the lemon and rinse the spinach.

Juice all the ingredients together.

Pour the juice into a glass and serve immediately.

## 125

### pear + avocado juice

SERVES 1

**375 g (13 oz) pears**

**75 g (2¾ oz) peeled and stoned avocado**

Remove the stalks from the pears, then roughly chop.

Put the pears in a blender or food processor with the avocado and blend until smooth.

Pour the juice into a glass and serve immediately.

## 126

### spiced root, spinach + orange juice

SERVES 2

**2 oranges**

**½ lemon**

**100 g (3½ oz) beetroot**

**100 g (3½ oz) carrots**

**100 g (3½ oz) celery**

**100 g (3½ oz) spinach**

**1-cm (½-inch) piece fresh root ginger**

Peel the oranges and lemon. Trim the beetroot and then scrub or peel.

Take the tops off the carrots and then scrub. Peel away any stringy bits from the celery. Rinse the spinach. Peel the ginger.

Juice all the ingredients together.

Pour the juice into glasses and serve immediately.

tip

This juice helps to lower blood pressure, aid digestion, boost the immune system and eliminate toxins. It is also great if your stress levels are high or if you are prone to migraines or nausea.

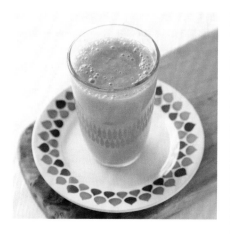

## carrot, beetroot, strawberry + orange
juice

SERVES 1

**100 g (3½ oz) beetroot**
**175 g (6 oz) carrots**
**125 g (4½ oz) strawberries**
**1 orange**
**ice cubes**

Trim the beetroot and then scrub or peel. Take the tops off the carrots and then scrub. Hull the strawberries. Peel the orange.

Juice all the prepared ingredients together.

Pour the juice over ice cubes in a glass and serve immediately.

 **tip**

Carrots, beetroot and oranges are all high in vitamin C, antioxidants and phytonutrients such as beta-carotene, and are also rich sources of potassium.

# 127

## mango + baobab
smoothie

SERVES 4

**1 orange**
**1 mango**
**1 small banana**
**3 ice cubes**
**1 tablespoon baobab powder**
**300 ml (10 fl oz) water**

Peel and then juice the orange. Peel and stone the mango, then roughly chop the flesh. Peel the banana, then roughly chop.

Transfer the orange juice to a blender or smoothie maker, add the mango, banana and the remaining ingredients and blend until smooth.

Pour the smoothie into glasses and serve immediately.

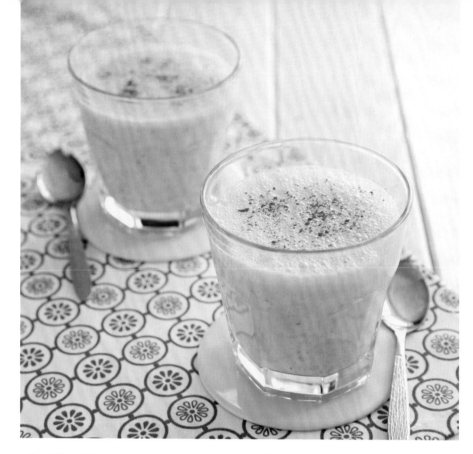

# 129

## orange, banana + muesli
### smoothie

SERVES 2

**2 oranges**

**1 banana**

**2 tablespoons muesli**

**300 ml (10 fl oz) milk**

**ground cinnamon,
to decorate**

Peel the oranges and then juice. Peel the banana, then roughly chop.

Transfer the orange juice to a blender or smoothie maker, add the banana, muesli and milk and blend until smooth.

Pour the smoothie into glasses, sprinkle with ground cinnamon and serve immediately.

# 130

## next time...

Add a nutty twist by replacing half the muesli with 1 tablespoon of nuts of your choice. Walnuts and pecans work particularly well.

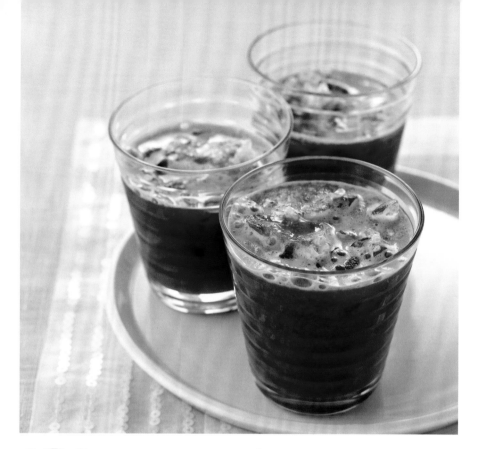

# 131

## carrot, beetroot + sweet potato juice

SERVES 1

**175 g (6 oz) sweet potato or yam**

**100 g (3½ oz) beetroot**

**175 g (6 oz) carrots**

**125 g (4½ oz) fennel, fronds reserved to decorate (optional)**

**ice cubes**

Peel the sweet potato or yam. Trim the beetroot and then scrub or peel. Take the tops off the carrots and then scrub. Trim the fennel.

Juice all the prepared ingredients together.

Pour the juice over ice cubes in a glass, decorate with fennel fronds, if liked, and serve immediately.

# 132

## apple, lemon + ginger
juice

SERVES 1

**3 apples**

**½ lemon**

**1 yellow pepper**

**2.5-cm (1-inch) piece fresh root ginger**

**ice cubes**

Remove the stalks from the apples. Peel the lemon half. Core and deseed the yellow pepper. Peel the ginger.

Juice all the prepared ingredients together.

Pour the juice over ice cubes in a glass and serve immediately.

# 133

## next time...

This juice is great diluted with a little hot (not boiling) water and served as a warm drink with a little ground cinnamon sprinkled over the top. If you like your drinks quite sour, add an extra squeeze of lemon juice.

# 134

## kale, cucumber + avocado smoothie

SERVES 1

**2 celery sticks**

**50 g (1¾ oz) kale**

**2-cm (¾-inch) piece fresh root ginger**

**1 garlic clove**

**1 cucumber**

**1 avocado**

**15 g (½ oz) parsley**

**sea salt and freshly ground black pepper**

**large handful of ice cubes**

Peel away any stringy bits from the celery. Cut any really woody stalks off the kale. Peel the ginger and garlic. Trim the cucumber and roughly chop. Peel and stone the avocado.

Juice the celery, kale and ginger together.

Transfer the juice to a blender or smoothie maker, add all the remaining ingredients and blend until smooth.

Pour the smoothie into a glass and serve immediately.

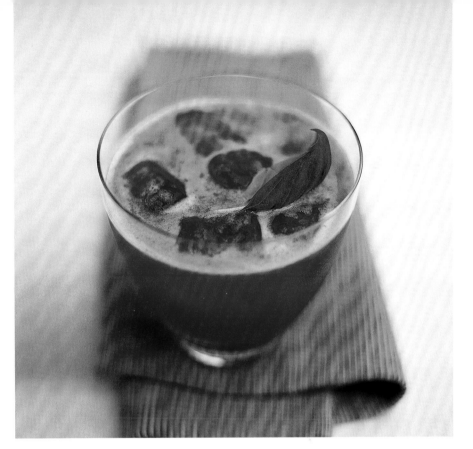

# 135

## strawberry, tomato + basil
juice

SERVES 1

**100 g (3½ oz) strawberries**

**200 g (7 oz) tomatoes**

**a few basil leaves, 1 reserved
for decoration**

**ice cubes**

Hull the strawberries. Juice the strawberries and tomatoes with the basil leaves.

Pour the juice over ice cubes in a glass, decorate with the reserved basil leaf and serve immediately.

### tip

This juice is full of phytonutrients including lycopene, which has been proven to have anti-cancer properties.

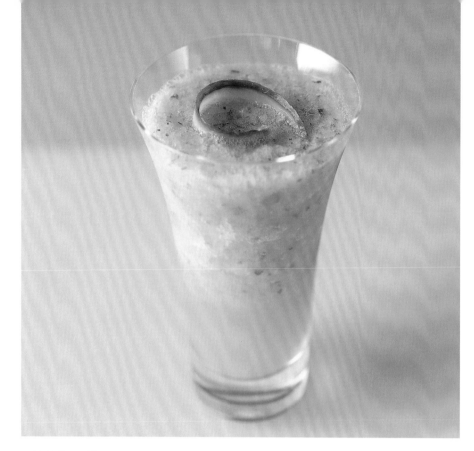

## 136

### cucumber, lemon + mint
smoothie

SERVES 1

**250 g (9 oz) cucumber, plus
an extra strip to decorate
(optional)**

**½ lemon**

**3-4 mint leaves**

**2-3 ice cubes**

Peel and roughly chop the cucumber. Squeeze the
juice from the lemon half.

Put the cucumber and lemon juice in a blender or
smoothie maker with the mint leaves and ice cubes
and blend briefly.

Pour the smoothie into a glass, decorate with
a cucumber strip, if liked, and serve immediately.

## 137
### next time...

Blend 1 cucumber, trimmed and roughly chopped,
with 150 ml (5 fl oz) grapefruit juice and a handful
of ice cubes in a blender or food processor to make
an ice-cold slushy drink.

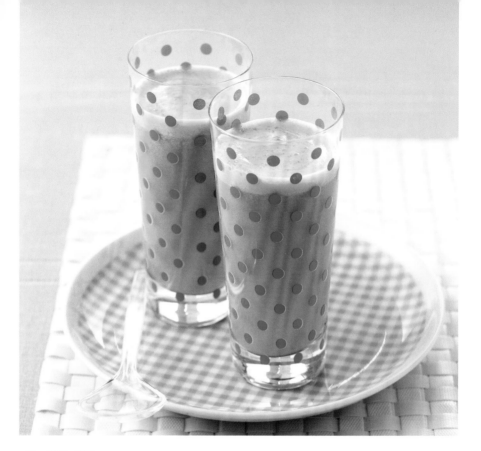

# 138

## melon, carrot + ginger juice

**SERVES 1**

**250 g (9 oz) cantaloupe melon**

**125 g (4½ oz) carrots**

**1 lime**

**1-cm (½-inch) piece fresh root ginger**

**ice cubes (optional)**

Peel the melon as close to the skin as possible and deseed, then roughly chop the flesh. Take the tops off the carrots and then scrub. Peel the lime and ginger.

Juice all the prepared ingredients together.

Pour the juice over ice cubes, if using, in a glass and serve immediately.

# 139

### next time...

Juice 2 carrots, tops trimmed and then scrubbed, with 1 orange, peeled, and 1 apple, stalk removed.

# 140

## lettuce, apple + carrot
juice

SERVES 1

**1 lemon**

**1 carrot**

**2 little gem lettuces**

**1 apple**

**1 teaspoon chia oil**

Grate the zest of the lemon and reserve. Peel the lemon. Take the top off the carrot and then scrub. Separate the lettuce leaves. Remove the stalk from the apple.

Juice the lemon with the carrot, lettuce and apple, taking care that the lettuce leaves do not clog the machine. Stir in the reserved grated lemon zest and chia oil. Serve immediately.

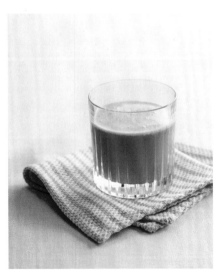

# 141

## mixed pepper juice

SERVES 1

**100 g (3½ oz) red pepper**

**100 g (3½ oz) yellow pepper**

**100 g (3½ oz) orange pepper**

**1 orange**

**1 tablespoon mint leaves**

**ice cubes**

Core and deseed all the peppers. Peel the orange.

Juice the peppers and orange together, then stir in the mint leaves.

Pour the juice over ice cubes in a glass and serve immediately.

This juice is great if you're run down and fighting a cold or flu. Peppers ward off infection and are natural painkillers.

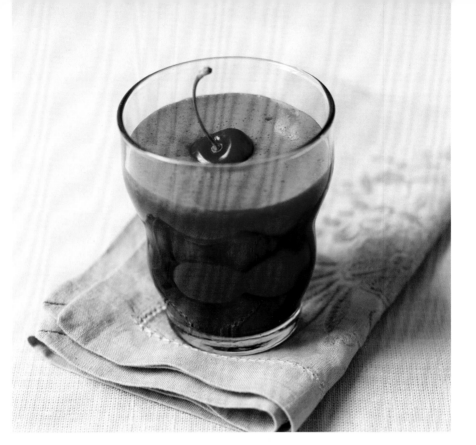

# 142

## beetroot, dark cherry + grape
juice

SERVES 1

**50 g (1¾ oz) beetroot**

**200 g (7 oz) sweet dark cherries, plus 1 extra to decorate**

**125 g (4½ oz) red seedless grapes**

Scrub or peel the beetroot. Stone the cherries.

Juice the beetroot, then the cherries and grapes.

Stir the juice, then pour into a glass, top with a cherry and serve immediately.

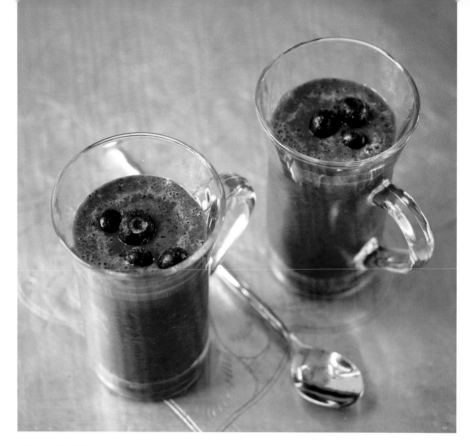

# 143

## beetroot + blueberry
### smoothie

SERVES 1

**50 g (1¾ oz) beetroot**

**125 g (4½ oz) blueberries, plus extra to decorate**

**90 ml (6 tablespoons) freshly squeezed orange juice**

**50 g (1¾ oz) low-fat natural yogurt**

**1 teaspoon agave syrup**

Scrub or peel the beetroot, then roughly chop. Put in a blender or smoothie maker, add all the remaining ingredients and blend until smooth.

Pour the smoothie into a glass, decorate with extra blueberries and serve immediately.

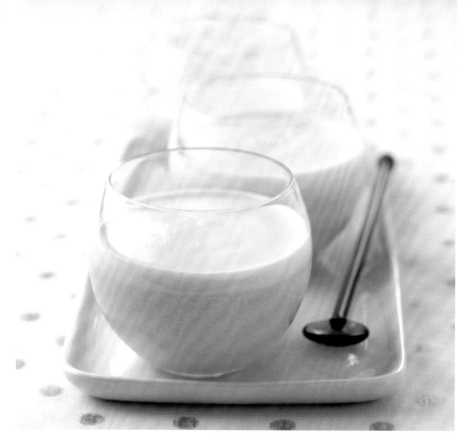

# 144

## melon, pineapple + apple
juice

SERVES 1

½ galia melon
¼ pineapple
3 green apples
ice cubes (optional)

Peel the melon as close to the skin as possible and deseed, then roughly chop the flesh. Cut the skin off the pineapple and remove the core if very tough. Remove the stalks from the apples.

Juice all the fruits together.

Pour the juice over ice cubes, if using, in a glass and serve immediately.

# 145

## next time...

Halve and stone 5 plums, then juice with 3 red apples, stalks removed. Serve over ice cubes.

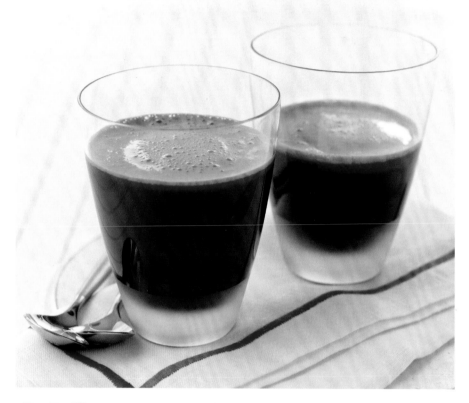

# 146

## red onion + beetroot
juice

SERVES 1

**250 g (9 oz) carrots**
**125 g (4½ oz) beetroot**
**125 g (4½ oz) red onion**
**1 garlic clove**
**125 g (4½ oz) watercress**

Take the tops off the carrots and then scrub. Trim the beetroot and then scrub or peel. Peel the red onion and garlic.

Juice all the prepared ingredients with the watercress.

Pour the juice into a glass and serve immediately.

# 147

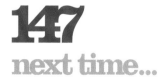
next time...

Juice 10 large carrots, tops trimmed and then scrubbed, and 4 large beetroots, trimmed and scrubbed or peeled, with a 2.5-cm (1-inch) piece fresh root ginger, peeled. Serve over ice cubes.

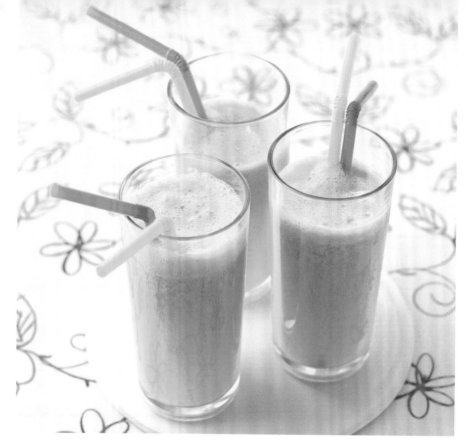

# 148

### orange, apple + pear
juice

SERVES 1

**2 oranges**

**1 red apple**

**1 pear**

**ice cubes (optional)**

**1 teaspoon clear honey
(optional)**

Peel the oranges. Remove the stalks from the apple and pear.

Juice all the fruits together.

Pour the juice over ice cubes, if using, in a glass, stir in the honey, if liked, and serve immediately.

# 149

## next time...

Juice 2 pears and 2 apples, stalks removed. Transfer the juice to a blender or food processor and blend with some ice cubes to make a slushy drink.

**97**

**150**

**151**

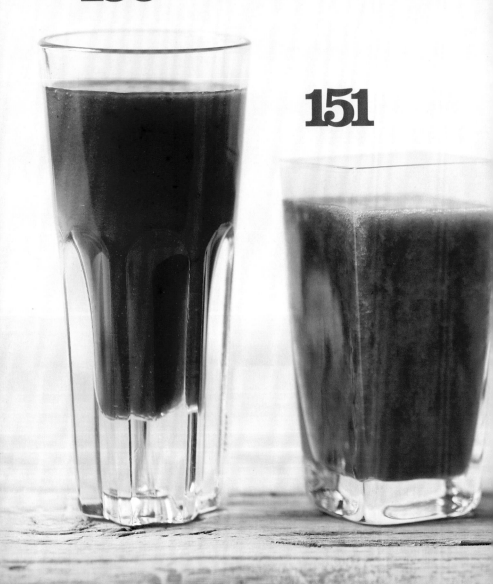

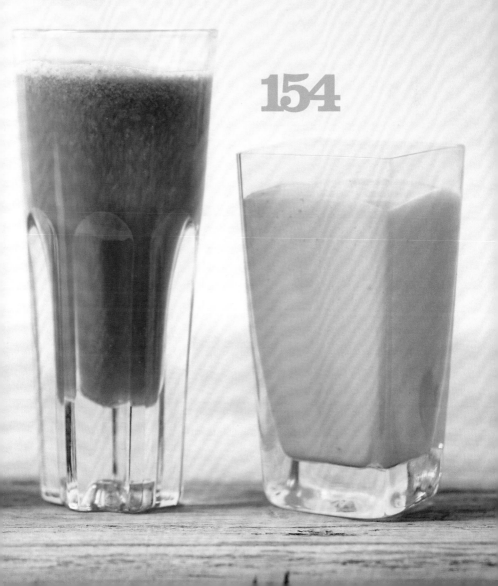

153

154

# 150

## pineapple + blackcurrant smoothie

SERVES 1

½ pineapple

1 banana

30 g (1 oz) fresh or frozen (defrosted) blackcurrants removed from their stalks

1 tablespoon coconut milk

Cut the skin off the pineapple and remove the core if very tough, then roughly chop. Peel the banana, then roughly chop.

Juice the pineapple and blackcurrants together.

Transfer the juice to a blender or smoothie maker, add the banana and coconut milk and blend until smooth.

Pour the smoothie into a glass and serve immediately.

# 151

## pineapple, grapefruit + plum juice

SERVES 1

¼ pineapple

3 plums

1 small red grapefruit

Cut the skin off the pineapple and remove the core if very tough. Halve and stone the plums. Peel the grapefruit.

Juice all the fruits together.

Pour the juice into a glass and serve immediately.

# 152

## gingered mango juice

SERVES 1

2-cm (¾-inch) piece fresh root ginger

2 mangoes

2 apples

ice cubes

Peel the ginger. Peel and stone the mangoes. Juice the ginger with the mangoes and apples.

Pour the juice into a glass over ice cubes and serve immediately.

## 153

# kiwifruit + cucumber
## juice

SERVES 1

**2 kiwifruits**

**½ small cucumber**

**75 g (2¾ oz) red seedless grapes**

**1 teaspoon agave syrup (optional)**

Peel the kiwifruits and trim the cucumber.

Juice the kiwifruits, cucumber and grapes together, then stir in the agave syrup to sweeten, if liked.

Pour the juice into a glass and serve immediately.

## 154

# mango + coconut milk
## smoothie

SERVES 1

**1 apple**

**½ large banana**

**75 ml (2½ fl oz) coconut milk**

**50 g (1¾ oz) natural coconut milk yogurt**

**150 g (5½ oz) frozen mango chunks**

**2 tablespoons water**

Remove the stalk from the apple and then juice. Peel the banana.

Transfer the juice to a blender or smoothie maker, add the banana and the remaining ingredients and blend until smooth.

Pour the smoothie into a glass and serve immediately.

tip

You can use 75 ml (2½ fl oz) apple juice instead of juicing the apple.

# 155

## wild rose infusion

SERVES 1

**100 g (3½ oz) freshly picked rosehips**
**200 ml (7 fl oz) boiling water**
**2 crisp dessert apples**
**ice cubes**
**wild rose petals, to decorate**

Put the rosehips in a food processor and process until finely chopped.

Turn the rosehips into a small saucepan and add the measured boiling water. Cover and simmer gently for 10 minutes, then leave to cool.

Remove the stalks from the apples and then juice.

Strain the rosehip juice into the apple juice.

Pour the infusion over ice cubes in a glass, decorate with rose petals and serve immediately.

**tip**

Wild roses provide an abundant, free supply of nutrient-rich rosehips, which are packed with vitamin C, a powerful antioxidant essential for natural immunity and energy.

# 156

## breakfast smoothie

SERVES 2

**1 tablespoon pomegranate juice**
**1 small banana, chopped**
**300 ml (10 fl oz) soya milk**
**1 tablespoon almonds**
**1 tablespoon rolled oats**
**½ teaspoon honey**
**½ tablespoon ground flax seeds**
**2 tablespoons natural yogurt**

Place all the ingredients in a blender and blend until smooth and creamy.

Pour into glasses and serve immediately.

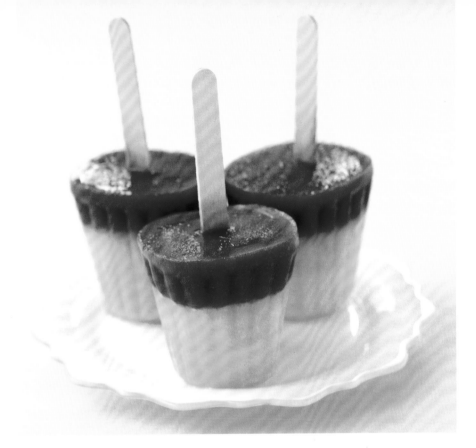

# 157

## apple, peach + strawberry
### lollies

MAKES 3–4 LOLLIES

**2 peaches**

**300 ml (10 fl oz) still mineral water**

**1 red apple**

**125 g (4½ oz) strawberries**

Halve and stone the peaches and then juice.

Stir one-third of the measured mineral water into the peach juice, then spoon into 3–4 lolly moulds. Freeze until just set.

Remove the stalk from the apple and then juice. Stir another third of the measured mineral water into the apple juice and pour over the frozen peach mixture. Freeze until just set.

Hull the strawberries and then juice. Stir the remaining measured mineral water into the strawberry juice, pour over the frozen apple mixture and freeze until set.

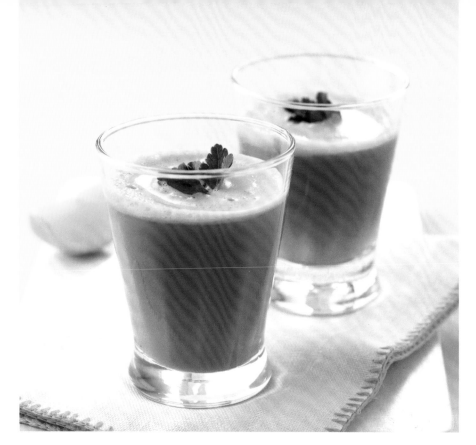

# 158

## carrot, parsnip + sweet potato juice

SERVES 1

**175 g (6 oz) celery**

**175 g (6 oz) carrots**

**175 g (6 oz) parsnip**

**175 g (6 oz) sweet potato**

**1 garlic clove**

**handful of parsley, plus an extra sprig to decorate (optional)**

**2-3 ice cubes**

**lemon wedge, to decorate**

Peel away any stringy bits from the celery. Take the tops off the carrots and then scrub. Peel the parsnip, sweet potato and garlic.

Juice all the vegetables, garlic and parsley together.

Transfer the juice to a blender or food processor, add the ice cubes and blend briefly.

Pour the juice into a glass, decorate with a lemon wedge and a parsley sprig, if liked, and serve immediately.

# 159

## blueberry, beetroot + baobab smoothie

SERVES 1

**1 small beetroot**

**1 small banana**

**200 g (7 oz) blueberries**

**300 ml (10 fl oz) water**

**1 tablespoon baobab powder**

**3 ice cubes**

Trim the beetroot and then scrub or peel. Peel the banana, then roughly chop.

Juice the beetroot.

Transfer the juice to a blender or smoothie maker, add the banana and all the remaining ingredients and blend until smooth.

Pour the smoothie into a glass and serve immediately.

# 160

## banana, oat + honey shake

SERVES 1

**1 small banana**

**25 g (1 oz) porridge oats**

**125 g (4½ oz) natural yogurt**

**125 ml (4 fl oz) semi-skimmed milk**

**1 teaspoon clear honey, plus extra to decorate**

**pinch of ground cinnamon**

Peel the banana, then roughly chop. Put in a blender or smoothie maker, add the oats, yogurt, milk, honey and cinnamon and blend until smooth.

Pour the smoothie into a glass, drizzle some honey on top and serve immediately.

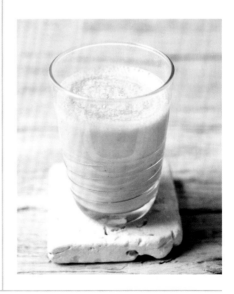

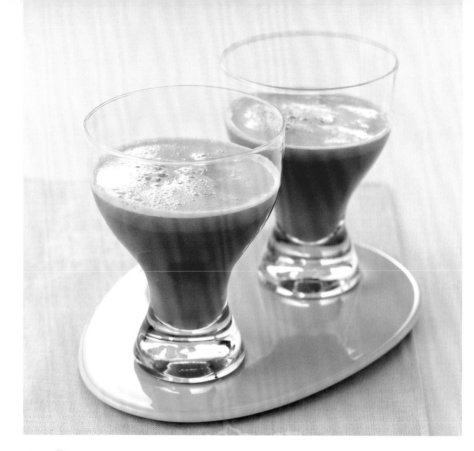

# 161

## carrot, fennel + ginger juice

SERVES 1

**300 g (10½ oz) carrots**

**75 g (2¾ oz) celery**

**2.5-cm (1-inch) piece fresh root ginger**

**50 g (1¾ oz) fennel, plus extra strips to decorate (optional)**

**1 tablespoon spirulina powder (optional)**

Take the tops off the carrots and then scrub. Peel away any stringy bits from the celery. Peel the ginger.

Juice the carrots, celery and ginger with the fennel and spirulina, if using. Pour the juice into a glass and serve immediately.

Both carrot and fennel are effective detoxifiers and good for restoring fluid balance because of their high potassium content.

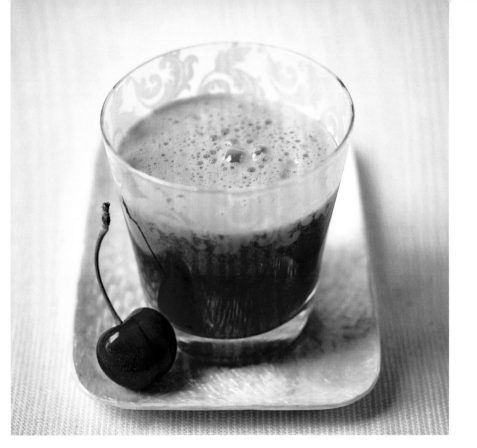

# 162

## apple + cherry juice

SERVES 1

**3 apples**

**150 g (5½ oz) red cherries**

Remove the stalks from the apples and stone the cherries.

Juice the apples and cherries together.

Pour the juice into a glass and serve immediately.

# 163

### next time...

Peel and roughly chop 3 kiwifruits, then juice with 2 large oranges, peeled and segmented.

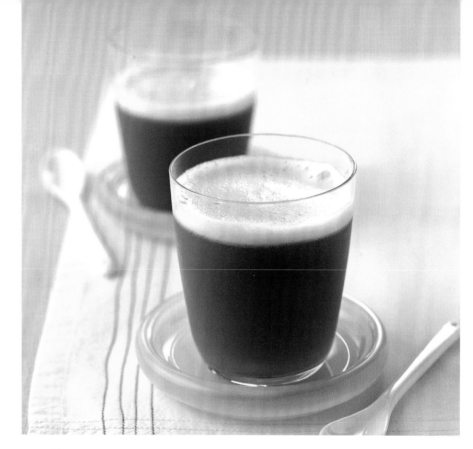

# 164

## Jerusalem artichoke, celery + celeriac juice

**SERVES 1**

**100 g (3½ oz) celeriac**

**100 g (3½ oz) Jerusalem artichokes**

**100 g (3½ oz) celery**

**small bunch of mint**

**2–3 ice cubes**

Peel the celeriac and cut into chunks. Scrub the Jerusalem artichokes. Peel away any stringy bits from the celery. Pull the mint leaves off their stalks.

Juice the vegetables with the mint, alternating the mint leaves with the other ingredients to make sure that the leaves do not clog the machine.

Transfer the juice to a blender or food processor, add the ice cubes and blend briefly.

Pour the juice into a glass and serve immediately.

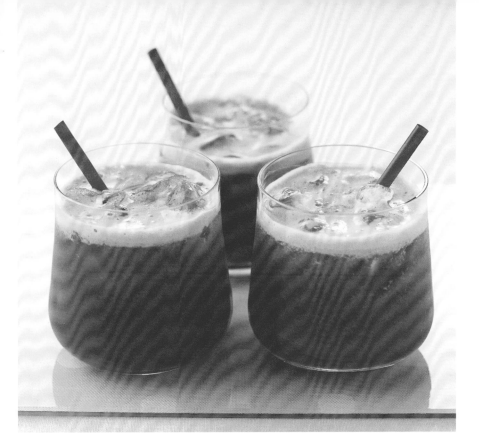

# 165

## strawberry, redcurrant + orange juice

SERVES 1

**100 g (3½ oz) strawberries**

**75 g (2¾ oz) redcurrants, plus extra to decorate (optional)**

**½ orange**

**125 ml (4 fl oz) still mineral water**

**½ teaspoon clear honey**

**ice cubes**

Hull the strawberries. Remove the stalks from the redcurrants. Peel the orange.

Juice all the fruits together, then stir in the measured mineral water and honey.

Pour the juice into a glass, add some ice cubes and decorate with extra redcurrants, if liked.

To make this juice into lollies, pour into lolly moulds after stirring in the honey and freeze.

## 166

# beetroot, apple + mint
juice

SERVES 1

**75 g (2¾ oz) beetroot**
**3 apples**
**8 mint leaves**

Trim the beetroot and then scrub or peel. Remove the stalks from the apples.

Juice the beetroot and apples with the mint.

Pour into a glass and serve immediately.

## 167

# lavender tea

SERVES 1

**3 lavender sprigs**
**½ teaspoon mild clear honey**
**200 ml (7 fl oz) boiling water**

Put the lavender sprigs in a cup with their stalk ends uppermost so that they can easily be lifted out.

Add the honey and measured boiling water to the cup and leave to infuse for 4–5 minutes before serving.

## 168

# blackberry + grape
smoothie

SERVES 1

**400 g (14 oz) purple seedless grapes or 300 ml (10 fl oz) purple grape juice**
**125 g (4½ oz) fresh or frozen blackberries**
**3 tablespoons live natural yogurt**

If using fresh grapes, juice them.

Transfer the grape juice, or ready-made grape juice, to a blender or smoothie maker, add the remaining ingredients and blend until smooth.

Pour the smoothie into a glass and serve immediately.

**tip**

Blackberries and purple grapes contain high levels of fluid-balancing potassium and essential bioflavonoids, while the addition of live natural yogurt boosts intestinal flora and calcium intake.

## 169

### five citrus juice

SERVES 1

**1 clementine**
**1 grapefruit**
**1 orange**
**1 lemon**
**1 lime**
**ice cubes**

Peel all the citrus fruits, then juice them together.

Pour the juice over ice cubes in a glass and serve immediately.

### green herb, apple + celery juice

SERVES 1

**2 green apples (such as Granny Smith)**
**1 celery stick**
**¼ cucumber**
**5 g (⅛ oz) coriander**
**5 g (⅛ oz) basil**

Remove the stalks from the apples. Peel away any stringy bits from the celery.

Juice all the ingredients together.

Pour the juice into a glass and serve immediately.

## 171

### aniseedy melon + mandarin infusion

SERVES 1

**3 whole star anise**
**½ teaspoon clear honey**
**150 ml (5 fl oz) water**
**150 g (5½ oz) cantaloupe melon**
**2 mandarins or 1 small orange**

Put the star anise and honey in a small saucepan with the measured water and bring slowly to the boil. Cover and simmer very gently for 5 minutes.

Meanwhile, cut a long wedge from the melon and reserve. Peel the remainder as close to the skin as possible and deseed, then roughly chop the flesh. Peel the mandarins or orange.

Juice the fruits together.

Pour the juice into a glass, then stir in the strained anise syrup. Serve warm or chilled, decorated with the melon wedge.

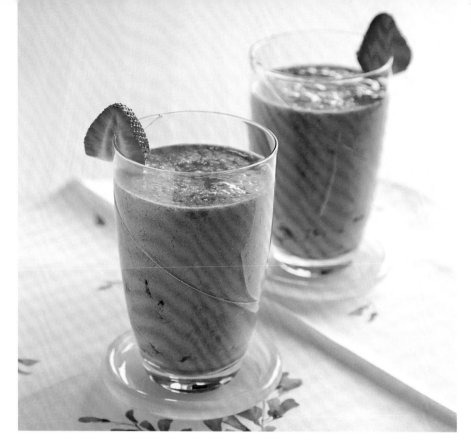

## 172

## berry, beetroot + banana
smoothie

SERVES 2

**1 beetroot**

**1 banana**

**85 g (3 oz) strawberries, plus extra slices to decorate**

**60 g (2¼ oz) raspberries**

**1 tablespoon flaked almonds**

**300 ml (10 fl oz) milk**

Trim the beetroot and then scrub or peel. Peel the banana, then roughly chop. Hull the strawberries.

Juice the beetroot. Transfer the beetroot juice to a blender or smoothie maker, add the banana, berries, almonds and milk and blend until smooth.

Pour the smoothie into glasses, decorate with extra strawberry slices and serve immediately.

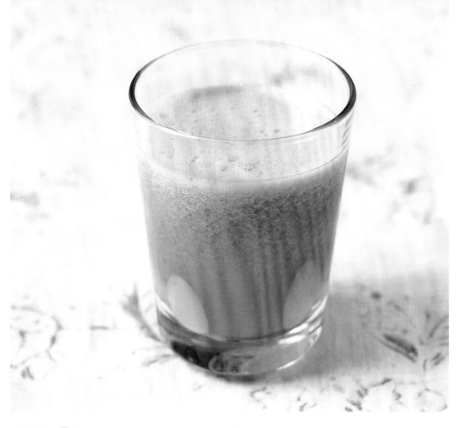

# 173

## cantaloupe, pear
## + grape juice

SERVES 1

SERVES 1

½ cantaloupe or other
    orange-fleshed melon

1 pear

75 g (2¾ oz) green seedless
    grapes

1 teaspoon freshly squeezed
    lime juice

Peel the melon as close to the skin as possible and deseed, then roughly chop. Remove the stalk from the pear and core.

Juice the melon, pear and grapes together, then stir in the lime juice.

Pour the juice into a glass and serve immediately.

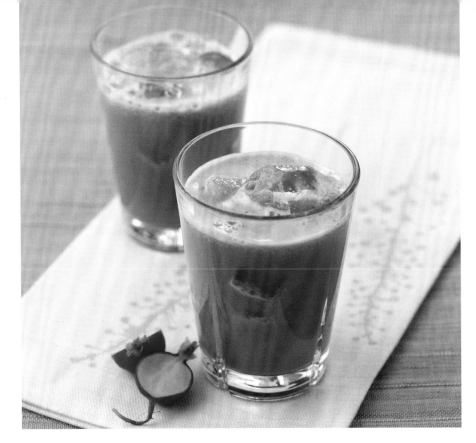

# 174

## carrot, radish + cucumber
juice

SERVES 1

**100 g (3½ oz) potato**

**100 g (3½ oz) carrots**

**100 g (3½ oz) radishes, plus
extra slices to decorate
(optional)**

**100 g (3½ oz) cucumber**

**ice cubes**

Peel the potato. Take the tops off the carrots and then scrub. Trim the radishes and cucumber.

Juice all the prepared ingredients together.

Transfer the juice to a blender or food processor, add a couple of ice cubes and blend briefly.

Pour the juice over ice cubes in a glass, decorate with radish slices, if liked, and serve immediately.

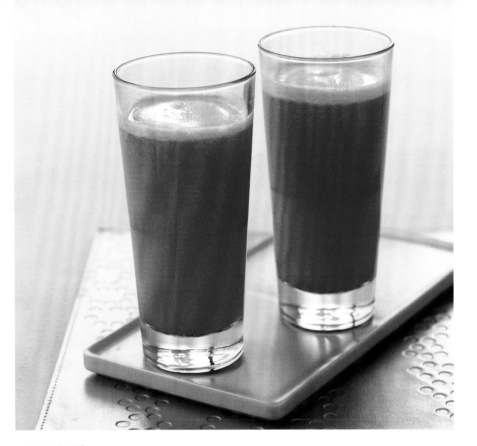

# 175

## orange + raspberry juice

**SERVES 1**

**2 large oranges**

**175 g (6 oz) raspberries**

**250 ml (9 fl oz) still mineral water**

**ice cubes (optional)**

Peel the oranges.

Juice the oranges and raspberries together, then stir in the measured mineral water.

Pour the juice over ice cubes, if using, in glasses and serve immediately.

## 176

# fig, mango + date
## smoothie

SERVES 1

**2 figs**
**½ mango**
**1–2 dates**
**25 g (1 oz) romaine lettuce leaves**
**150 ml (5 fl oz) coconut water**
**juice of ¾ lime**

Remove the stalks from the figs. Peel and chop the mango. Stone the dates. Tear the lettuce leaves.

Put all the ingredients in a blender or smoothie maker and blend until smooth.

Pour the smoothie into a glass and serve immediately.

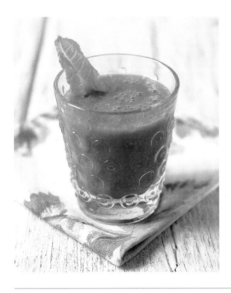

## 177

# chocolate orange
## smoothie

SERVES 1

**1 orange**
**½ banana**
**100 g (3½ oz) blueberries**
**1–2 teaspoons cocoa powder**
**½ teaspoon grated orange zest**
**50–75ml (2–2½ fl oz) almond milk**

Peel the oranges and then juice. Peel the banana, then roughly chop.

Transfer the orange juice to a blender or smoothie maker, add the banana, blueberries, cocoa and orange zest and blend until smooth.

Blend in the almond milk to achieve your desired consistency.

Pour the smoothie into a glass and serve immediately.

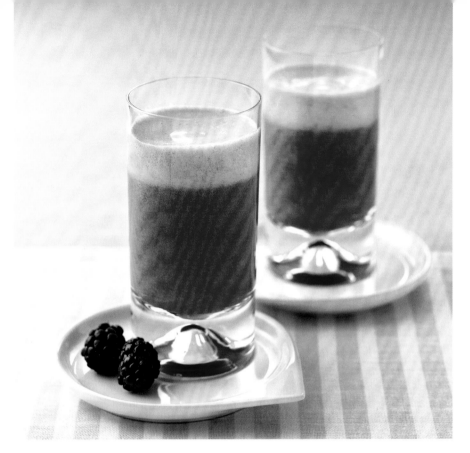

## apple, blackberry + melon
juice

SERVES 1

**100 g (3½ oz) cantaloupe melon**

**100 g (3½ oz) fresh or frozen blackberries, plus extra to decorate**

**100 ml (3½ fl oz) apple juice**

**2–3 ice cubes**

Peel the melon as close to the skin as possible and deseed, then roughly chop. Juice the blackberries with the melon.

Transfer the juice to a food processor or blender, add the apple juice and a couple of ice cubes and process briefly.

Pour the juice into a glass, decorate with a few blackberries and serve immediately.

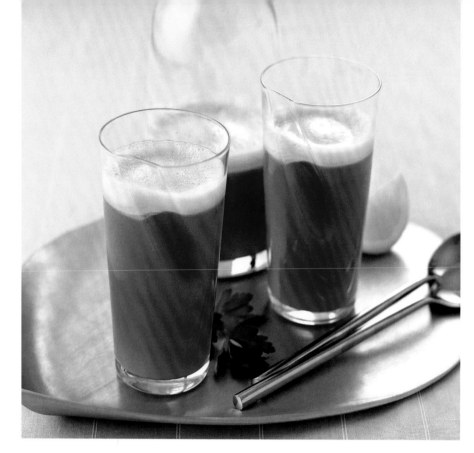

# 179

## carrot, chicory + celery juice

**SERVES 1**

**175 g (6 oz) carrots**

**125 g (4½ oz) celery**

**125 g (4½ oz) chicory**

**2–3 ice cubes**

**lemon wedges, to decorate**

Take the tops off the carrots and then scrub. Peel away any stringy bits from the celery. Separate the chicory leaves.

Juice the carrots, celery and chicory together.

Transfer the juice to a blender or food processor, add the ice cubes and blend briefly.

Pour the juice into a glass, decorate with lemon wedges, if liked, and serve immediately.

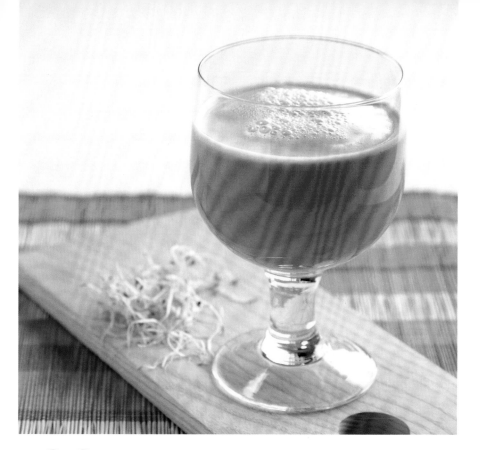

# 180

## apple, ginger + alfalfa juice

SERVES 1

**1 lemon**

**2-cm (¾-inch) piece fresh root ginger**

**1 garlic clove**

**1 apple**

**1 carrot**

**2 celery sticks**

**100 g (3½ oz) alfalfa sprouts**

Peel the lemon, ginger and garlic. Remove the stalk from the apple. Take the top off the carrot and then scrub. Peel away any stringy bits from the celery. Rinse the alfalfa sprouts.

Juice all the ingredients together.

Pour the juice into a glass and serve immediately.

# 181

## mint + cardamom green tea

SERVES 1

**5 cardamom pods**

**large pinch of cumin seeds**

**3 mint sprigs, plus extra leaves to decorate**

**1 green tea bag**

**200 ml (7 fl oz) boiling water**

**clear honey, to taste**

Lightly crush the cardamom pods and cumin seeds using a pestle and mortar. Add the mint sprigs and bruise the leaves to release the natural oils.

Turn the mint and spices into a small jug or teapot along with the teabag and pour over the measured boiling water.

Leave to infuse for 4 minutes, then strain into a cup. Add a little honey to taste, decorate with extra mint leaves and serve hot.

**tip**

Cardamom pods are great for the digestive system.

# 182

## citrus, cucumber + ginger fizz

SERVES 1

**1 lemon**

**1 lime**

**2-cm (¾-inch) piece fresh root ginger**

**½ cucumber**

**sparkling mineral water, for topping up**

Peel the lemon, lime and ginger. Trim the cucumber.

Juice all the ingredients together.

Pour the juice into a glass and top up with sparkling mineral water.

# 183

## mint lassi cooler

SERVES 1

**150 g (5½ oz) natural yogurt**

**¼ cucumber**

**8 mint leaves, plus extra sprigs to decorate**

**2 ice cubes**

Put all the ingredients in a blender or smoothie maker and blend until smooth.

Pour into a glass, decorate with mint sprigs and serve immediately.

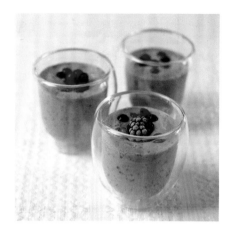

# 184

## berry + apple yogurt
smoothie

SERVES 1

**2 apples**
**50 g (1¾ oz) frozen mixed summer**
**berries, plus extra to decorate**
**125 g (4½ oz) natural yogurt**

Remove the stalks from the apples and then juice.

Transfer the juice to a blender or smoothie maker, add the berries and yogurt and blend until smooth.

Pour the smoothie into a glass, decorate with extra berries and serve immediately.

**tip**

If you are in a hurry, use 125 ml (4 fl oz) cloudy apple juice instead of juicing the apples.

# 185

## blackcurrant + almond
smoothie

SERVES 4

**250 g (9 oz) blackcurrants**
**750 g (1 lb 10 oz) natural yogurt**
**1 teaspoon natural almond essence**
**1–2 tablespoons agave nectar, to taste**
**toasted almonds, to decorate**

Remove the stalks from the blackcurrants, put in a blender or smoothie maker and blend to a purée.

Add the yogurt, almond essence and agave nectar, according to taste, to a large bowl and beat together. Gently fold in the blackcurrant purée.

Spoon the smoothie into glasses, decorate with toasted almonds and serve immediately.

# 186

## plum + strawberry juice

SERVES 1

**2 plums**
**2 sweet apples**
**1 orange**
**50 g (1¾ oz) strawberries**

Halve and stone the plums. Remove the stalks from the apples. Peel the orange and hull the strawberries.

Juice all the ingredients together.

Pour the juice into a glass and serve immediately.

# 187

## kiwifruit, strawberry + nectarine juice

SERVES 1

**2 nectarines**
**2 kiwifruits**
**150 g (5½ oz) strawberries**

Halve and stone the nectarines. Peel the kiwifruits. Hull the strawberries.

Juice all the fruits together.

Pour the juice into a glass and serve immediately.

# 188

## rhubarb + watermelon juice

SERVES 1

**200 g (7 oz) watermelon**
**1 small rhubarb stick**
**1 celery stick**
**8 mint leaves, plus an extra sprig to decorate**

Peel the watermelon as close to the skin as possible and deseed, then roughly chop the flesh. Trim the rhubarb and peel away any stringy bits from the celery.

Juice the mint, rhubarb and celery, followed by the watermelon.

Pour the juice into a glass, decorate with a mint sprig and serve immediately.

### tip

If your juicer is a very heavy-duty one, you can just scrub the watermelon skin clean and include it in the juice, rather than peeling.

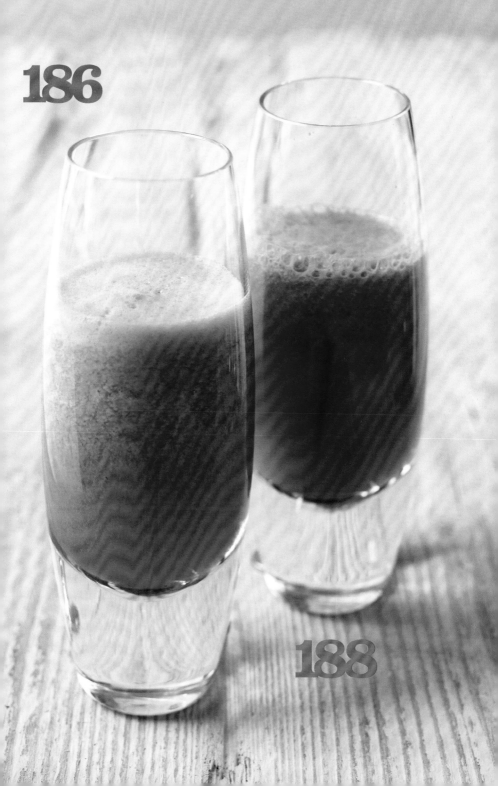

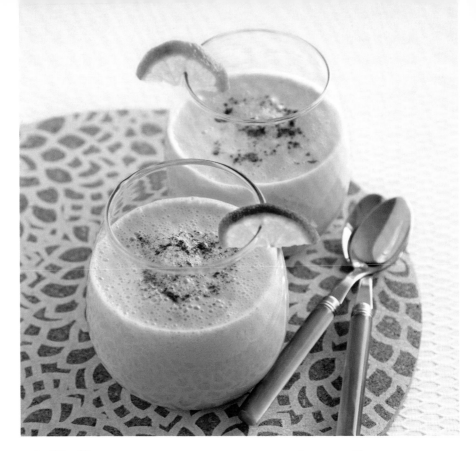

# 189

## papaya, apricot + lime hemp milk smoothie

**SERVES 2**

**1 papaya**

**1 apricot**

**1 lime, plus extra slices to decorate**

**400 ml (14 fl oz) hemp milk**

**1 teaspoon chia oil**

**¼ teaspoon ground cinnamon**

Peel and deseed the papaya, then roughly chop the flesh. Halve and stone the apricot. Peel and then juice the lime.

Transfer the lime juice to a blender or smoothie maker, add all the remaining ingredients and blend until smooth.

Pour the smoothie into glasses, decorate each glass with a lime slice and serve immediately.

# 190

## next time...

For a refreshing minty twist, add 10–12 mint leaves to the blender or smoothie maker with the other ingredients.

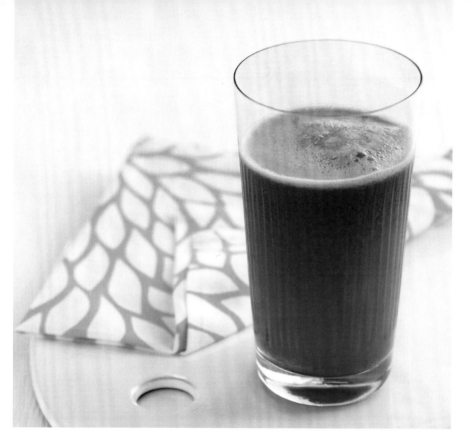

## 191

### celery, spinach + apple
juice

SERVES 1

**60 g (2¼ oz) spinach**
**1 apple**
**2 celery sticks**

Rinse the spinach. Remove the stalk from the apple. Peel away any stringy bits from the celery.

Juice all the ingredients together.

Pour the juice into a glass and serve immediately.

## 192
### next time...

Stir in ½ teaspoon green powder (such as wheatgrass, spirulina or chlorella) and 1 teaspoon avocado oil for an extra power boost.

# 193

## blueberry + grapefruit smoothie

SERVES 1

**125 g (4½ oz) grapefruit**
**250 g (9 oz) apples**
**2.5-cm (1-inch) piece fresh root ginger**
**125 g (4½ oz) blueberries**

Peel the grapefruit. Remove the stalks from the apples. Peel the ginger, then roughly chop.

Juice the grapefruit and apples together.

Transfer the juice to a blender or smoothie maker, add the ginger and blueberries and blend until smooth.

Pour the smoothie into a glass and serve immediately.

# 194

## peanut butter + banana smoothie

SERVES 4

**½ lime**
**150g (5 oz) banana**
**1 tablespoon peanut butter**
**300 ml (½ pint) almond milk**
**grated nutmeg, to decorate**

Peel and then juice the lime. Peel the banana, then roughly chop.

Transfer the lime juice and banana to a food processor or blender, add the peanut butter and almond milk and process until smooth.

Pour the smoothie into glasses, sprinkle with a large pinch of nutmeg and serve immediately.

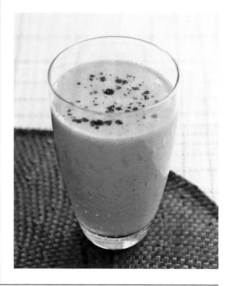

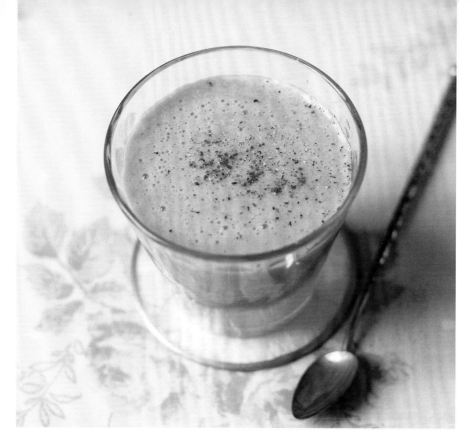

# 195

## spiced apple + pear juice

SERVES 1

**2 apples**

**1 large pear**

**½ lemon**

**60 g (2¼ oz) green seedless grapes**

**pinch of ground cinnamon**

**pinch of ground nutmeg**

**pinch of ground cloves**

**ice cubes**

Remove the stalks from the apples and the pear. Peel the lemon.

Juice all the fruits together, then stir in the spices.

Pour the juice over ice cubes in a glass and serve immediately. Alternatively, for a winter juice, warm the juice through in a saucepan, pour into a heatproof glass and serve warm.

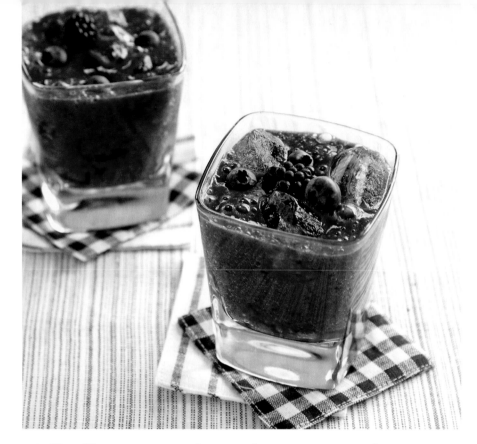

# 196

## berry, banana + apple
### smoothie

SERVES 2

**2 apples**

**1 large banana**

**250 g (9 oz) mixed berries,
plus extra to decorate**

**ice cubes**

Remove the stalks from apples. Peel the banana, then roughly chop. Juice the apples.

Transfer the apple juice to a blender or smoothie maker, add the banana and mixed berries and blend until smooth, adding a little water, if necessary, if you want a looser consistency.

Pour the smoothie over ice cubes in glasses, decorate with a few extra berries and serve.

# 197
## next time...

Go green by adding 60 g (2¼ oz) spinach, rinsed, to the juicer with the apple.

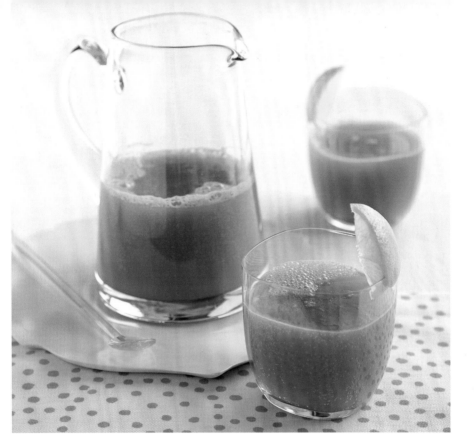

# 198

## spinach + cucumber lemonade

SERVES 2

**2 lemons, plus extra wedges to decorate**

**1 cucumber**

**30 g (1 oz) spinach**

**sparkling mineral water, for topping up**

Peel the lemons. Trim the cucumber. Rinse the spinach.

Juice the lemons with the cucumber and spinach.

Pour the juice into a glass and top up with sparkling mineral water. Decorate with a lemon wedge and serve immediately.

# 199
## next time...

Replace the spinach with 2 oranges, peeled, for a more citrusy version of this lemonade.

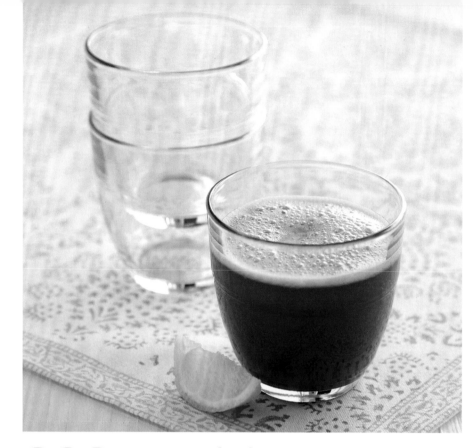

# 200

## spicy lemon, apple + parsley juice

SERVES 1

**2 lemons**

**1-cm (½-inch) piece fresh horseradish root**

**1 apple**

**15 g (½ oz) parsley**

Peel the lemons and horseradish. Remove the stalk from the apple.

Juice all the ingredients together.

Pour the juice into a glass and serve immediately.

# 201
## next time...

Juice 2 lemons, peeled, and a 1-cm (½-inch) piece fresh horseradish root, peeled, pour into a cup and top up with boiling water.

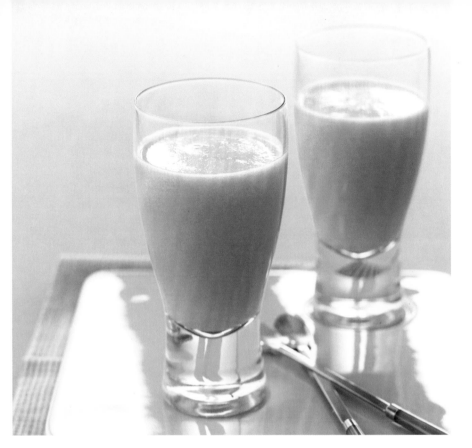

# 202

## apple, mango + passionfruit
juice

SERVES 1

**1 mango**

**2 passionfruits**

**3 apples, preferably red, plus extra slices to decorate (optional)**

**ice cubes**

Peel and stone the mango. Cut the passionfruits in half, scoop out the seeds and pulp and discard the seeds. Remove the stalks from the apples.

Juice all the fruits together.

Pour the juice over ice cubes in a glass, decorate with apple slices, if liked, and serve immediately.

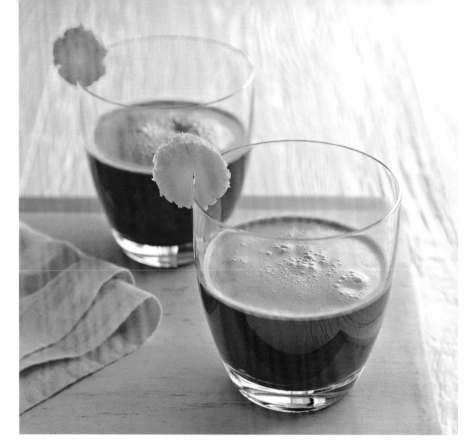

# 203

### citrus beetroot juice

SERVES 1

**1 orange**

**1 beetroot**

**1 large carrot, plus an extra
slice to decorate**

**½ cucumber**

Peel the orange. Trim the beetroot and then scrub
or peel. Take the top off the carrot and then scrub.
Trim the cucumber.

Juice all the ingredients together.

Pour the juice into a glass, decorate with carrot
slices and serve immediately.

# 204
### next time...

To spice this juice up, add a 2-cm (¾-inch) piece
fresh root ginger, peeled, to the juicer with the
other ingredients.

# 205

## broccoli + apple juice

SERVES 1

**½ head of broccoli**
**2 large or 3 smaller apples**
**2-cm (¾-inch) piece fresh root ginger**

Trim the broccoli. Remove the stalks from the apples. Peel the ginger.

Juice all the ingredients together.

Pour the juice into a glass and serve immediately.

# 206

## next time...

Swap the broccoli for 40 g (1½ oz) spinach, rinsed.

# 207

## peach + carrot juice

SERVES 1

**3 peaches**
**1 carrot**
**2-cm (¾-inch) piece fresh root ginger**

Halve and stone the peaches. Take the top off the carrot and then scrub. Peel the ginger.

Juice all the ingredients together.

Pour the juice into a glass and serve immediately.

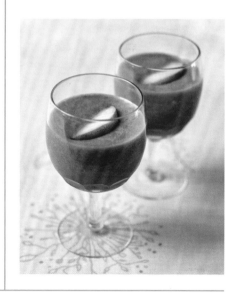

# 208

## beetroot, celery + coriander juice

SERVES 1

**1 large beetroot**
**2 celery sticks**
**15 g (½ oz) coriander leaves**
**large pinch of ground turmeric**
**freshly ground black pepper**

Trim the beetroot and then scrub or peel. Peel away any stringy bits from the celery.

Juice the beetroot, celery and coriander together, then whisk in the turmeric and season to taste with black pepper.

Pour the juice into a glass and serve immediately.

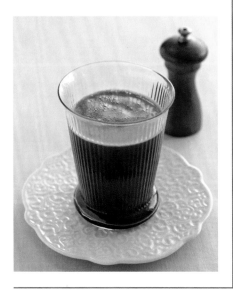

# 209

## asparagus + ginger juice

SERVES 1

**1 apple**
**2-cm (¾-inch) piece fresh root ginger**
**½ cucumber**
**6 asparagus spears**
**ice cubes**

Remove the stalk from the apple. Peel the ginger. Trim the cucumber.

Juice the apple, ginger, cucumber and asparagus together.

Pour the juice into a glass over ice and serve immediately.

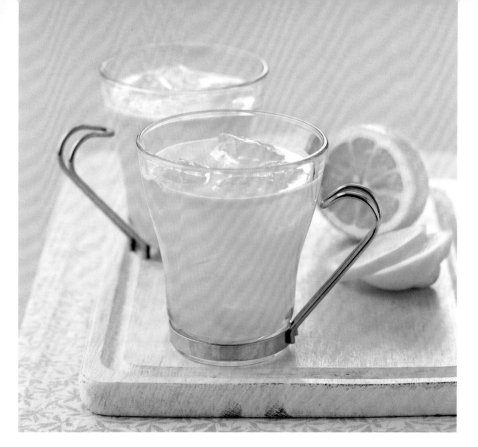

# 210

### fennel + camomile juice

SERVES 1

**1 lemon, plus extra slices to decorate (optional)**

**150 g (5½ oz) fennel**

**100 ml (3½ fl oz) camomile tea, chilled**

**ice cubes**

Peel the lemon and trim the fennel.

Juice the lemon and fennel together, then stir in the chilled camomile tea.

Pour the juice over ice cubes in a glass, decorate with lemon slices, if liked, and serve immediately.

# 211

## next time...

Juice ½ lemon with 200 g (7 oz) lettuce. Mix the juice with 100 ml (3½ fl oz) chilled camomile tea. Pour over ice cubes in a glass and decorate with a slice of lemon.

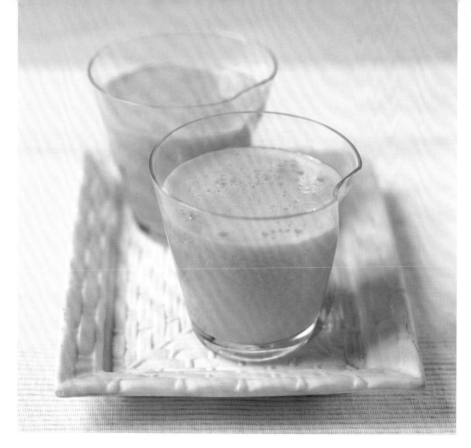

# 212

## kumquat + pear juice

SERVES 1

**2 pears**

**2-cm (¾-inch) piece fresh root ginger**

**10 kumquats**

**ice cubes**

Remove the stalks from the pears. Peel the ginger.

Juice the pears and kumquats with the ginger.

Pour the juice over ice cubes in a glass and serve immediately.

 **tip**

There is no need to peel the kumquats – just wash them well.

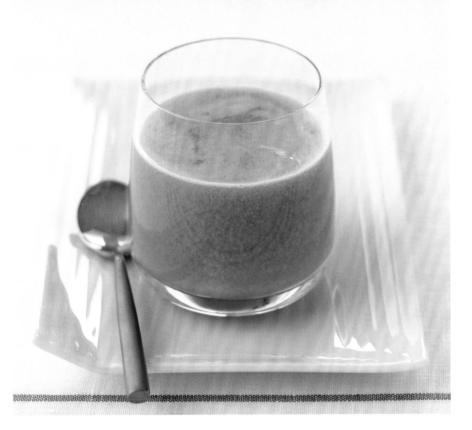

# 213

**lettuce + kiwifruit** juice

SERVES 1

**100 g (3½ oz) kiwifruits, plus extra slices to decorate (optional)**

**200 g (7 oz) lettuce**

**ice cubes (optional)**

Peel the kiwifruits. Separate the lettuce leaves.

Juice the kiwifruits and lettuce together, alternating the ingredients so that the lettuce leaves do not clog the machine.

Pour the juice over ice cubes, if using, in a glass, decorate with kiwifruit slices, if liked, and serve immediately.

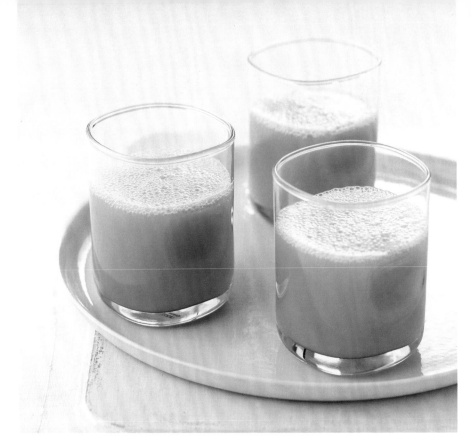

# 214

## lettuce, grape + ginger
juice

SERVES 1

**200 g (7 oz) lettuce**

**2.5-cm (1-inch) piece fresh root ginger**

**200 g (7 oz) green seedless grapes, plus extra to decorate (optional)**

**ice cubes (optional)**

Separate the lettuce leaves and peel the ginger.

Juice the grapes and lettuce with the ginger, alternating the ingredients so that the lettuce leaves do not clog the machine.

Pour the juice into a glass, decorate with a few grapes, if liked, and serve immediately.

Alternatively, for a creamier drink, transfer the juice to a blender or food processor, add a couple of ice cubes and blend briefly.

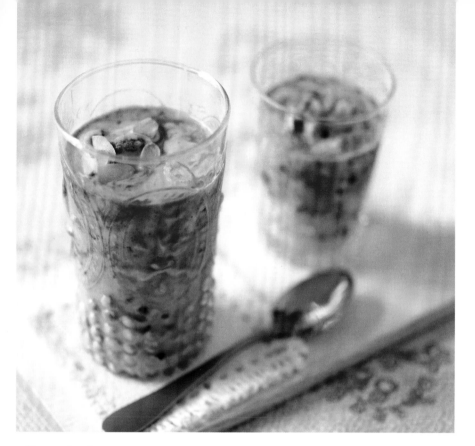

# 215

## mixed berry + vanilla fromage frais smoothie

**SERVES 4**

**3 tablespoons crème de cassis or spiced red fruit cordial**

**250 g (9 oz) mixed frozen berries**

**500 g (1 lb 2 oz) fat-free fromage frais**

**400 ml (14 fl oz) milk**

**1 vanilla pod, split in half lengthways**

**toasted flaked almonds, to decorate**

Put the crème de cassis or cordial in a saucepan over a low heat and gently heat, then add the berries. Stir, cover and cook for about 5 minutes or until the fruit has defrosted and is beginning to collapse. Remove from the heat and leave to cool completely.

Transfer most of the berry mixture with all the fromage frais and milk to a blender or smoothie maker and blend until smooth.

Scrape in the seeds from the vanilla pod and blend briefly to combine.

Fold the reserved berries into the fromage frais mixture until just combined. Spoon into glasses, decorate with toasted flaked almonds and serve.

**139**

# 216

## exotic fruit + coconut cream smoothie

SERVES 4

**5 tablespoons coconut cream**

**250 g (9 oz) frozen mixed exotic fruit**

**1 tablespoon freshly squeezed lime juice**

**500 g (1 lb 2 oz) fromage frais**

**250 g (9 oz) fat-free mango yogurt**

**toasted coconut flakes, to decorate**

Put 3 tablespoons of the coconut cream in a saucepan over a low heat and gently heat, then add the frozen exotic fruit and lime juice. Stir, cover and cook for about 5 minutes or until the fruit has defrosted and is beginning to collapse. Remove the pan from the heat and leave to cool completely.

Transfer the fruit mixture to a blender or smoothie maker and blend until smooth.

Mix the fromage frais with the remaining coconut cream and the mango yogurt, then fold into the fruit purée.

Spoon into glasses, sprinkle with toasted coconut flakes and serve immediately.

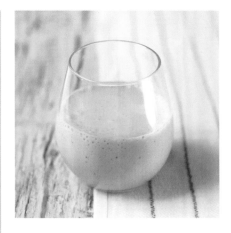

# 217

## banana + almond smoothie

SERVES 1

**1 banana**

**200 ml (7 fl oz) almond milk**

**1 tablespoon almond butter**

**few drops of natural almond essence (optional)**

Peel and slice the banana, put it in a freezerproof container and freeze for at least 2 hours or overnight.

Transfer the frozen banana to a blender or smoothie maker, add all the remaining ingredients and blend until smooth.

Pour the smoothie into a glass and serve immediately.

# 218

## pear, lychee + spinach juice

SERVES 1

**10 fresh lychees**
**2 pears**
**25 g (1 oz) spinach**
**2-cm (¾-inch) piece fresh root ginger**
**½ lime**

Peel and stone the lychees. Remove the stalks from the pears. Rinse the spinach. Peel the ginger.

Juice the prepared ingredients with the unpeeled lime half.

Pour the juice into a glass and serve immediately.

# 219

## next time...

Swap the lychees for 10 rambutans, peeled and stoned, and use 25 g (1 oz) lamb's lettuce instead of spinach.

# 220

## cranberry, apple + ginger juice

SERVES 1

**2 apples**
**2-cm (¾-inch) piece fresh root ginger**
**150 g (5½ oz) cranberries**
**1 teaspoon agave syrup (optional)**

Remove the stalks from the apples. Peel the ginger.

Juice the apples and cranberries with the ginger, then stir in the agave syrup to sweeten, if liked.

Pour the juice into a glass and serve immediately.

# 221

## mango + coconut juice

SERVES 1

**3 mangoes**
**200 ml (7 fl oz) coconut water**
**ice cubes**

Peel and stone the mangoes, then roughly chop the flesh.

Put the mango in a blender or smoothie maker and blend until smooth.

Stir in the coconut water, then pour over ice cubes in a glass and serve immediately.

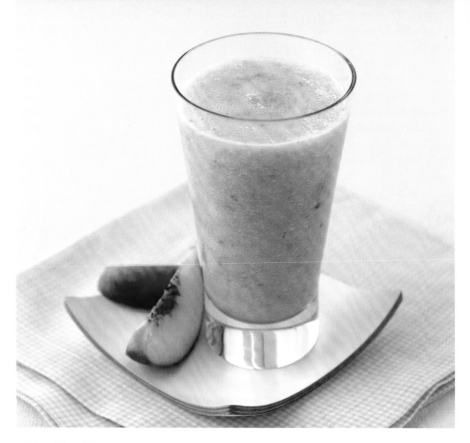

## 222

### apple, apricot + peach juice

SERVES 1

**3 apricots**

**1 peach, plus extra slices to
  decorate (optional)**

**2 apples**

**ice cubes**

Halve and stone the apricots and peach. Remove
the stalks from the apples.

Juice all the fruits together.

Transfer the juice to a blender or food processor,
add a few ice cubes and blend briefly.

Pour the juice into a glass, decorate with peach
slices, if liked, and serve immediately.

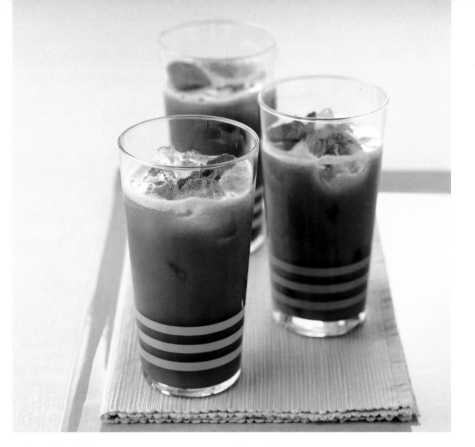

## 223

### parsnip, green pepper + watercress juice

SERVES 1

**175 g (6 oz) green pepper**
**175 g (6 oz) cucumber**
**175 g (6 oz) parsnip**
**100 g (3½ oz) watercress**
**ice cubes**
**chopped mint, to decorate**

Core and deseed the green pepper. Trim the cucumber. Peel the parsnip.

Juice the prepared ingredients with the watercress.

Pour the juice over ice cubes in a glass, decorate with a sprinkling of chopped mint and serve immediately.

## 224

### next time...

Juice 40 g (1½ oz) watercress with 3 pears, stalks removed. This simple juice is highly nutritious.

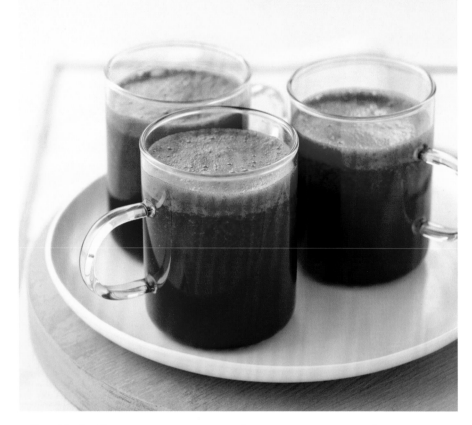

# 225

## strawberry, carrot + beetroot
juice

SERVES 1

**250 g (9 oz) carrots**

**125 g (4½ oz) beetroot**

**1 orange**

**125 g (4½ oz) strawberries,
plus extra to decorate
(optional)**

**ice cubes**

Take the tops off the carrots and then scrub.
Trim the beetroot and then scrub or peel. Peel the
orange. Hull the strawberries.

Juice the carrots, beetroot and orange together.

Transfer the juice to a blender or food processor,
add the strawberries and a few ice cubes and blend
until smooth.

Pour the juice into a glass, decorate with a
strawberry, if liked, and serve immediately.

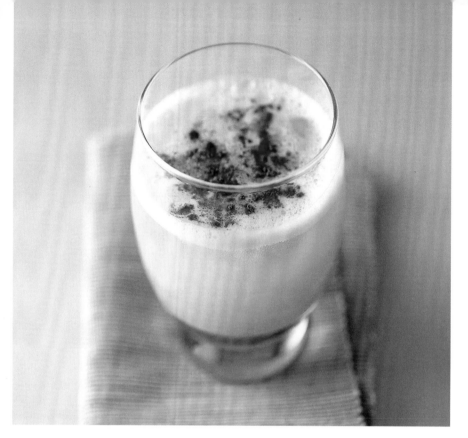

# 226

## cabbage, apple + cinnamon
juice

SERVES 1

**200 g (7 oz) green cabbage**

**50 g (1¾ oz) apple**

**2–3 ice cubes**

**large pinch of ground cinnamon, plus extra to decorate**

Trim the cabbage and then juice with the apple.

Transfer the juice to a blender or food processor, add the ice cubes and the cinnamon and blend briefly.

Pour the juice into a glass, decorate with extra cinnamon and serve immediately.

# 227

**next time...**

Juice 125 g (4½ oz) red cabbage with ½ orange and a handful of seedless red grapes to make a bright and only slightly sweet drink.

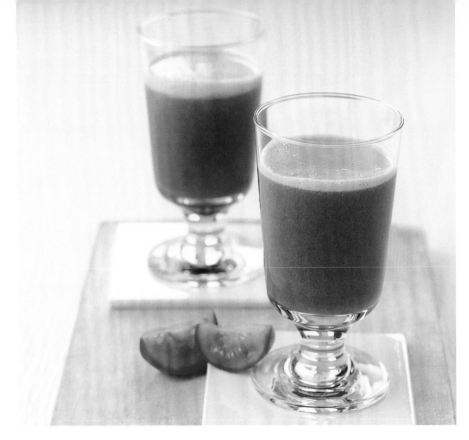

# 228

## seven vegetable juice

SERVES 1

**50 g (1¾ oz) green pepper**

**50 g (1¾ oz) celery**

**90 g (3¼ oz) carrots**

**25 g (1 oz) onion**

**25 g (1 oz) spinach**

**90 g (3¼ oz) cucumber**

**50 g (1¾ oz) tomatoes, plus extra quarters to decorate (optional)**

**sea salt and freshly ground black pepper**

Core and deseed the green pepper. Peel away any stringy bits from the celery. Take the tops off the carrots and then scrub. Peel the onion. Rinse the spinach. Trim the cucumber.

Juice all the ingredients except the seasoning together, taking care that the spinach leaves do not clog the machine.

Pour the juice into a glass and season with sea salt and black pepper. Decorate with tomato quarters, if liked, and serve immediately.

## 229

# cinnamon apple iced tea

SERVES 1

**4 apples**
**200 ml (7 fl oz) tea, chilled**
**large pinch of ground cinnamon**
**small handful of crushed ice**
**cinnamon stick, to decorate**

Remove the stalks from the apples and then juice.

Stir in the chilled tea, then add the ground cinnamon and stir to combine.

Pour the tea over crushed ice in a glass and serve with the cinnamon stick for stirring.

## 230

# tomato, orange + celery juice

SERVES 2

**2 oranges**
**2 celery sticks, plus an extra 2 leafy sticks to decorate**
**2 carrots**
**4 tomatoes**
**ice cubes**

Peel the oranges. Peel away any stringy bits from the celery. Take the tops off the carrots and then scrub. Juice the prepared ingredients with the tomatoes.

Pour the juice over ice cubes in glasses, add a leafy celery stick stirrer to each glass and serve immediately.

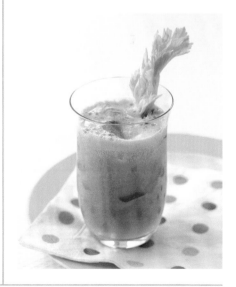

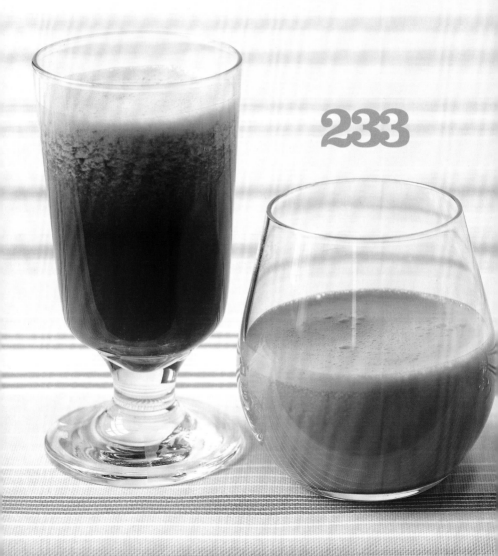

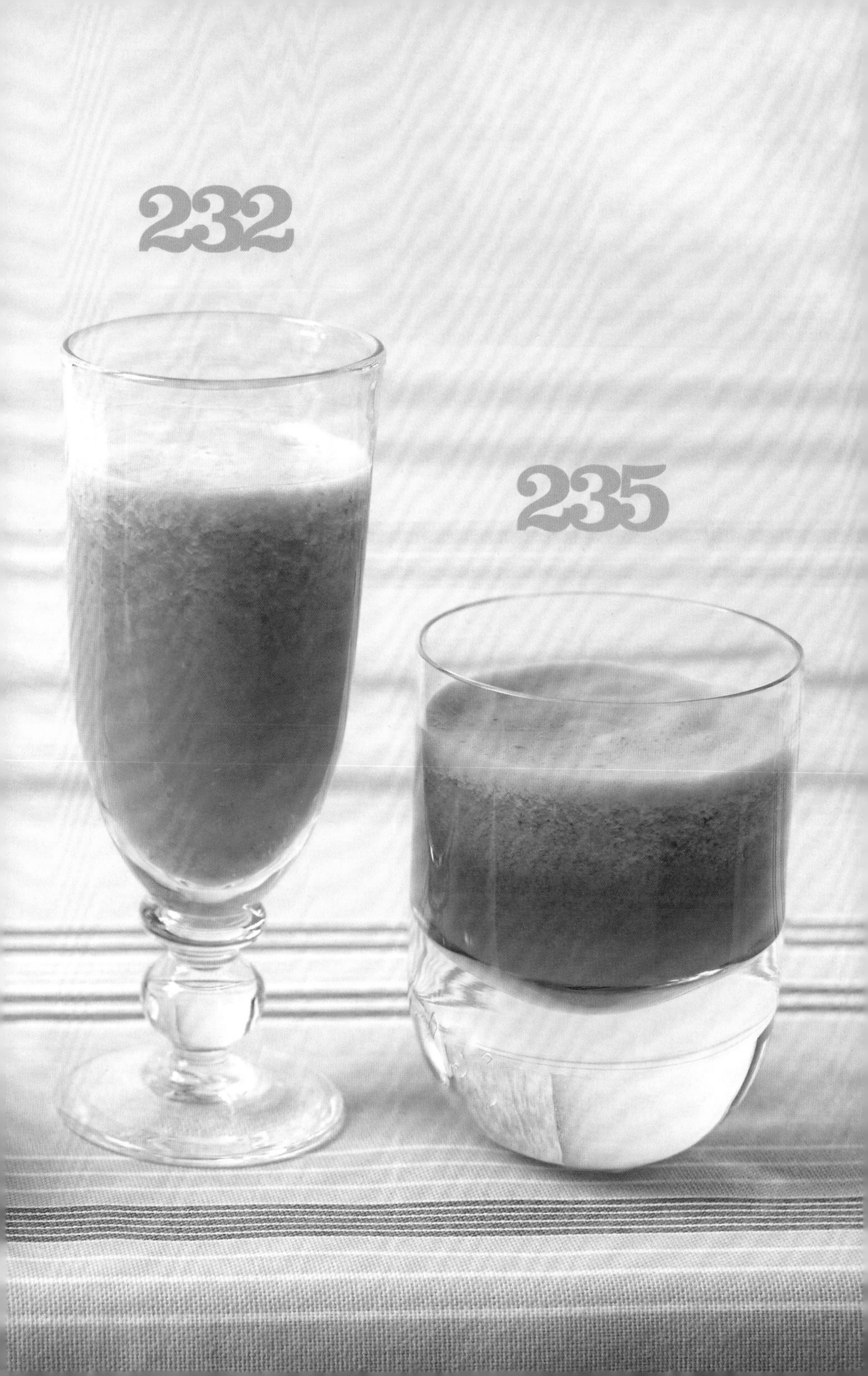
232
235

## 231

### red cabbage, melon + orange juice

SERVES 1

**2 oranges**
**½ galia or cantaloupe melon**
**¼ red cabbage**
**25 g (1 oz) fennel**

Peel the oranges. Peel the melon as close to the skin as possible and deseed, then roughly chop.

Juice all the ingredients together.

Pour the juice into a glass and serve immediately.

## 232

### broccoli + pineapple juice

SERVES 1

**4 Tenderstem broccoli spears**
**1 apple**
**¼ pineapple**
**10 g (¼ oz) watercress**

Trim the broccoli. Remove the stalk from the apple. Cut the skin off the pineapple and remove the core if tough.

Juice all the ingredients together. Pour the juice into a glass and serve immediately.

## 233

### carrot, sweet potato + orange juice

SERVES 1

**2 oranges**
**1 carrot**
**150 g (5½ oz) sweet potato**
**juice of 1 lime**

Peel the oranges. Take the top off the carrot and then scrub. Scrub the sweet potato, removing any scabby bits.

Juice the oranges, carrot and sweet potato together, then stir in the lime juice.

Pour the juice into a glass and serve immediately.

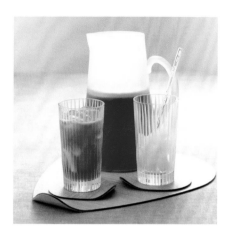

# 235

## apple, celery + coriander juice

SERVES 1

**4 celery sticks**
**2 apples**
**25 g (1 oz) kale**
**10 g (¼ oz) coriander leaves, plus extra to decorate**

Peel away any stringy bits from the celery. Remove the stalks from the apples. Cut any really woody stalks off the kale.

Juice all the ingredients together.

Pour the juice into a glass, decorate with a few extra coriander leaves and serve immediately.

# 234

## pear + cranberry juice

SERVES 1

**1 large pear**
**100 ml (3½ fl oz) cranberry juice**
**ice cubes**

Remove the stalk from the pear and then juice.

Mix the pear juice with the cranberry juice.

Pour the juice over ice cubes in a glass and serve immediately.

# 236

## fig, kiwifruit + nut
smoothie

SERVES 4

**2 kiwifruits**
**5 dried figs**
**300 ml (10 fl oz) almond milk**
**1 tablespoon protein powder**
**4 walnut halves**
**¼ teaspoon ground cinnamon**

Peel and then juice the kiwifruits. Remove the stalks from the figs, then roughly chop.

Transfer the kiwifruit juice to a blender or smoothie maker, add the figs and the remaining ingredients and blend until smooth. Pour the smoothie into glasses and serve immediately.

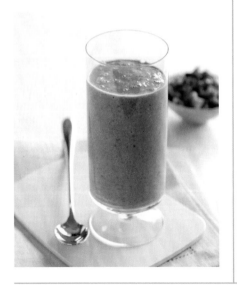

# 237

## pecan + yogurt
smoothie

SERVES 2

**50 g (1¾ oz) pecan nuts**
**250 g (9 oz) natural yogurt**
**300 ml (10 fl oz) fresh apple juice**
**clear honey, to taste**
**ice cubes**

Put the pecans in a blender or smoothie maker with a few tablespoons of the yogurt and process to a paste.

Add the remaining yogurt and the apple juice and blend again until well mixed. Sweeten to taste with honey.

Pour the smoothie over ice cubes in a glass and serve immediately.

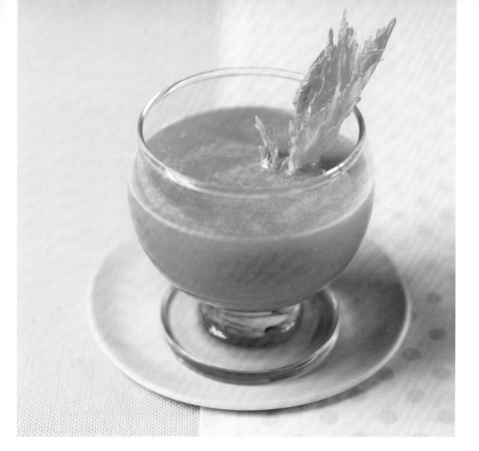

# 238

## orange, celery + mango
### smoothie

SERVES 1

**2 oranges**

**2 celery sticks, plus an extra leafy stick to decorate**

**1 carrot**

**½ large mango**

Peel the oranges. Peel away any stringy bits from the celery. Take the top off the carrot and then scrub. Peel the mango and roughly chop the flesh.

Juice the oranges, celery and carrot together.

Transfer the juice to a blender or smoothie maker, add the mango and blend until smooth, adding a little water if the consistency is too thick.

Pour the smoothie into a glass, add a leafy celery stick stirrer and serve immediately.

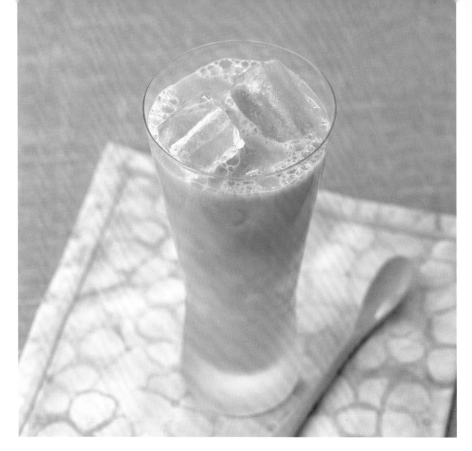

## 239

## pear, celery + ginger juice

SERVES 1

**100 g (3½ oz) pear**

**50 g (1¾ oz) celery**

**2.5-cm (1-inch) piece fresh root ginger**

**ice cubes**

Remove the stalk from the pear. Peel away any stringy bits from the celery. Peel the ginger.

Juice the pear, celery and ginger together.

Pour the juice over ice cubes in a glass and serve immediately.

Alternatively, transfer the juice to a blender or food processor and blend with 2–3 ice cubes, then pour into a glass and serve immediately.

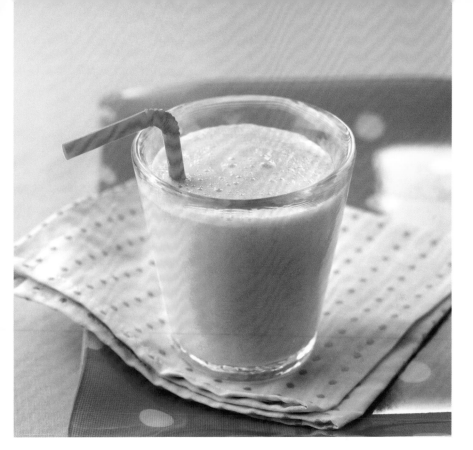

# 240

## pineapple, parsnip + carrot
smoothie

SERVES 2

**250 g (9 oz) pineapple, plus
extra wedges to decorate
(optional)**

**100 g (3½ oz) parsnip**

**100 g (3½ oz) carrots**

**75 ml (2½ fl oz) soya milk**

**ice cubes**

Cut the skin off the pineapple and remove the core
if very tough, then roughly chop the flesh. Peel the
parsnip. Remove the tops from the carrots and
then scrub.

Juice the pineapple, parsnip and carrots together.

Transfer the juice to a blender or smoothie maker,
add the soya milk and some ice cubes and blend
until smooth.

Pour the smoothie into glasses, decorate with
pineapple wedges, if liked, and serve immediately.

# 241

## cranberry + raspberry
smoothie

SERVES 1

**75 ml (2½ fl oz) pure cranberry juice**
**150 g (5½ oz) frozen raspberries**
**75 g (2¾ oz) natural yogurt**
**1 teaspoon agave syrup (optional)**

Put all the ingredients in a blender or smoothie maker and blend until smooth.

Pour the smoothie into a glass and serve immediately.

# 242

## baobab, banana +
## Greek yogurt smoothie

SERVES 1

**1 banana**
**125 ml (4 fl oz) semi-skimmed milk.**
**50 g (1¾ oz) natural Greek yogurt**
**1 teaspoon baobab powder**

Peel the banana, then roughly chop. Put in a blender or smoothie maker, add all the remaining ingredients and blend until smooth.

Pour the smoothie into a glass and serve immediately.

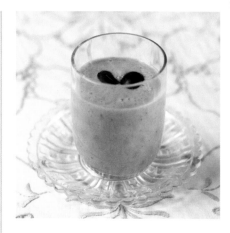

# 243

## fig + grape smoothie

SERVES 1

**2 figs**
**1 apple**
**½ banana**
**100 g (3½ oz) red seedless grapes, plus one extra grape, halved, to decorate**
**50 g (1¾ oz) natural yogurt**

Remove the stalks from the figs and apple. Peel the banana, then roughly chop.

Juice the apple and grapes together.

Transfer the juice to a blender or smoothie maker, add the figs, banana and yogurt and blend until smooth.

Pour the smoothie into a glass, decorate with grape halves and serve immediately.

## 244

# spicy roots + apple
## juice

SERVES 1

**1 parsnip**
**1 carrot**
**1 apple**
**2-cm (¾-inch) piece fresh root ginger**
**large pinch of ground turmeric**

Peel the parsnip. Take the top off the carrot and then scrub. Remove the stalk from the apple. Peel the ginger.

Juice all the ingredients except the turmeric together, then whisk in the turmeric.

Pour the juice into a glass and serve immediately.

## 245

# apricot, apple + orange
## juice

SERVES 1

**10 apricots**
**1 apple**
**1 orange**

Halve and stone the apricots. Remove the stalks from the apples. Peel the orange.

Juice all the fruits together.

Pour the juice into a glass and serve immediately.

## 246

# apricot, vanilla + honey
## smoothie

SERVES 1

**10 apricots**
**50 g (1¾ oz) natural yogurt**
**125 ml (4 fl oz) semi-skimmed milk**
**drop of vanilla extract**
**drizzle of clear honey**

Halve and stone the apricots. Put in a blender or smoothie maker, add all the remaining ingredients and blend until smooth.

Pour the smoothie into a glass and serve immediately.

## 247

### cabbage + pear juice

SERVES 1

**250 g (9 oz) pears**

**125 g (4½ oz) cabbage**

**50 g (1¾ oz) celery, plus an extra short stick to decorate (optional)**

**25 g (1 oz) watercress**

**ice cubes (optional)**

Remove the stalks from the pears. Trim the cabbage. Peel away any stringy bits from the celery.

Juice the prepared ingredients with the watercress.

Pour the juice over ice cubes, if using, in a glass and serve immediately with a short celery stick, if liked.

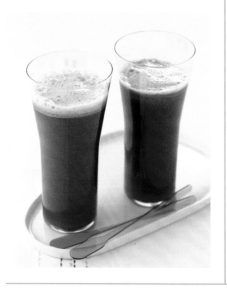

## 248

### banana + papaya
smoothie

SERVES 1

**1 banana**

**1 papaya**

**1 orange**

**300 ml (10 fl oz) apple juice**

**ice cubes**

Peel the banana, then roughly chop. Peel and deseed the papaya, then roughly chop the flesh. Peel and juice the orange.

Transfer the orange juice to a blender or food processor, add the banana, papaya, apple juice and a few ice cubes. Process until smooth.

Pour the smoothie into a glass and serve immediately.

## 249

### next time...

For a protein boost, add 2 tablespoons whey protein powder to the blender or smoothie maker with the other ingredients.

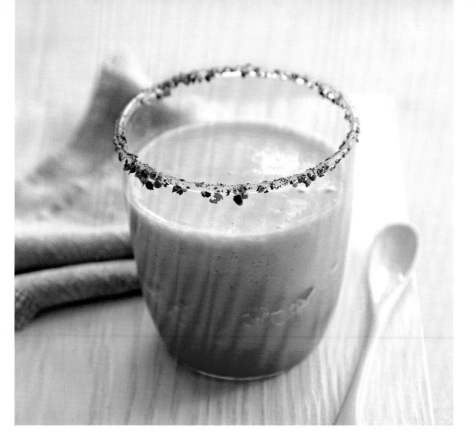

# 250

### sweet pepper juice

SERVES 1

**1 teaspoon ground mixed peppercorns**

**1 lime wedge**

**1 red pepper**

**20 red seedless grapes**

**2-3 ice cubes**

Spread the ground peppercorns on a small plate. Rub the rim of a glass with the lime wedge and dip the rim of the glass into the peppercorns to coat the rim.

Core and deseed the red pepper. Juice the red pepper and grapes together. Transfer the juice to a blender or food processor, add the ice cubes and blend briefly. Pour into the prepared glass and serve immediately.

# 251
## next time...

Core and deseed 1 red pepper. Juice the pepper with 1 apple and a 2-cm (¾-inch) piece peeled fresh root ginger. Serve with a dash of Tabasco.

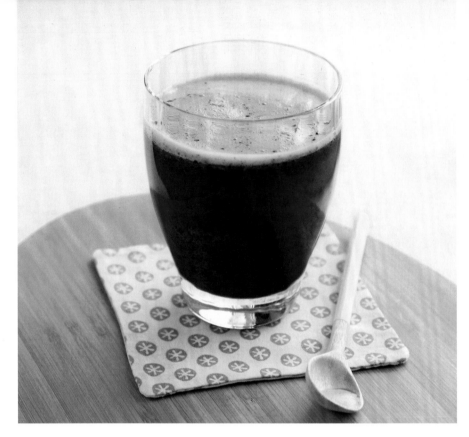

## 252

### leafy greens, cucumber + apple juice

SERVES 1

**1 little gem lettuce**

**2 celery sticks**

**½ cucumber**

**1 apple**

**30 g (1 oz) spinach**

**40 g (1½ oz) kale**

**½ teaspoon spirulina powder**

**1 teaspoon hemp seed oil**

**ice cubes**

Separate the lettuce leaves. Peel away any stringy bits from the celery. Trim the cucumber. Remove the stalk from the apple. Rinse the spinach. Cut any really woody stalks off the kale.

Juice all the ingredients together, then stir in the spirulina and hemp seed oil.

Pour the juice over ice cubes in a glass and serve immediately.

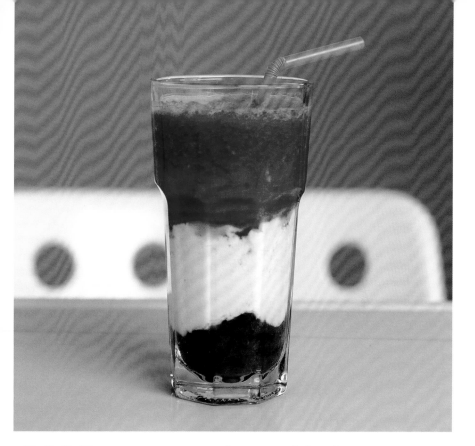

## 253

### raspberry + blueberry
smoothie

SERVES 1

**250 g (9 oz) raspberries**

**200 ml (7 fl oz) fresh apple juice**

**200 g (7 oz) blueberries**

**4 tablespoons Greek yogurt**

**100 ml (3½ fl oz) skimmed milk**

**1 tablespoon clear honey, or to taste**

**1 tablespoon wheatgerm (optional)**

Put the raspberries and half the apple juice in a blender or smoothie maker and blend to a purée. Pour into a jug.

Blend the blueberries with the remaining apple juice to a purée.

Mix the yogurt, milk, honey and wheatgerm, if using, together in a jug and add a spoonful of the raspberry purée.

Pour the blueberry purée into a tall glass. Carefully pour over the yogurt mixture, and then pour the raspberry purée over the surface of the yogurt. Serve chilled.

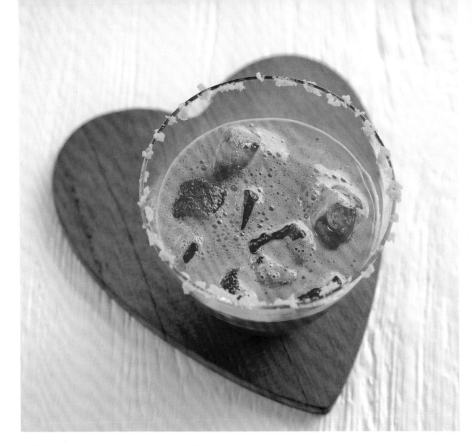

# 254

## beetroot, apple + orange
juice

SERVES 1

**1 beetroot**
**1 apple**
**1 orange**
**ice cubes**

Trim the beetroot and then scrub or peel. Remove the stalk from the apple. Grate the zest of the orange on to a plate. Peel the orange and then cut into wedges.

Rub the rim of a glass with an orange wedge, then dip the rim of the glass into the grated orange zest to coat the rim.

Juice the orange wedges, beetroot and apple together.

Pour the juice over ice cubes in the prepared glass and serve immediately.

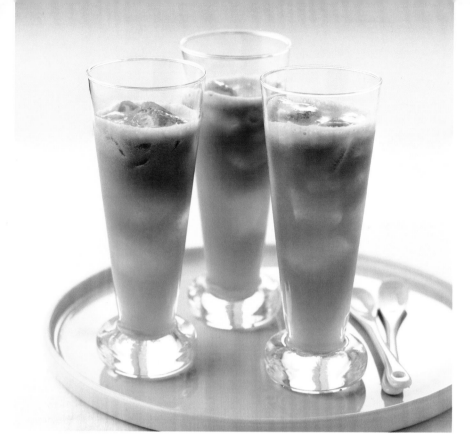

## 255

### spinach, celery + cucumber
juice

SERVES 1

**50 g (1¾ oz) green pepper**

**50 g (1¾ oz) celery**

**25 g (1 oz) spinach**

**100 g (3½ oz) cucumber**

**100 g (3½ oz) tomatoes**

**sea salt and freshly ground
    black pepper**

**ice cubes (optional)**

Core and deseed the green pepper. Peel away any stringy bits from the celery. Rinse the spinach. Trim the cucumber

Juice all the prepared vegetables and tomatoes together, then season to taste with sea salt and black pepper.

Pour the juice over ice cubes, if using, in a glass, and serve immediately.

## 256

## cashew nut +
## blueberry smoothie

SERVES 4

½ lime
100 g (3½ oz) blueberries
1 tablespoon cashew nut butter
300 g (10½ oz) low-fat live natural yogurt

Roughly peel and then juice the lime.

Transfer the lime juice and blueberries to a food processor or blender, add the cashew nut butter and yogurt and process until smooth.

Pour the smoothie into a glass and serve immediately.

## 257

## dandelion + mint
## infusion

SERVES 1

1 tablespoon dried dandelion leaves
handful of fresh mint leaves

Add the dandelion and mint leaves to a cafetière or teapot. Pour over freshly boiled water and leave to infuse for 10 minutes.

Pour into a cup and serve.

## 258

## tomato, cauliflower
## + carrot juice

SERVES 1

100 g (3½ oz) cauliflower
200 g (7 oz) carrots
1 large tomato

Trim the cauliflower and cut into chunks. Take the tops off the carrots and then scrub.

Juice all the ingredients together.

Pour the juice into a glass and serve immediately.

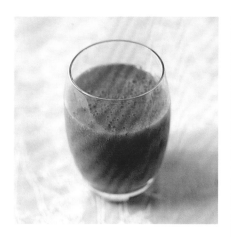

## 259

## orange + summer fruit
smoothie

SERVES 1

**2 oranges**
**75 g (2¾ oz) strawberries**
**75 g (2¾ oz) raspberries**

Peel the oranges and hull the strawberries. Put all the ingredients in a blender or smoothie maker and blend until smooth. Pour into a glass and serve immediately.

## 260

## next time...

Juice the strawberries with 2–3 apples, stalks removed, instead of the oranges.

## 261

## apple, cucumber
## + mint juice

SERVES 1

**2 sweet apples**
**½ cucumber**
**8 mint leaves**

Remove the stalks from the apples. Trim the cucumber.

Juice the apples and cucumber with the mint.

Pour the juice into a glass and serve immediately.

## 262

## next time...

Replace the 2 apples with ¾ honeydew melon, peeled as close to the skin as possible and deseeded, then roughly chopped.

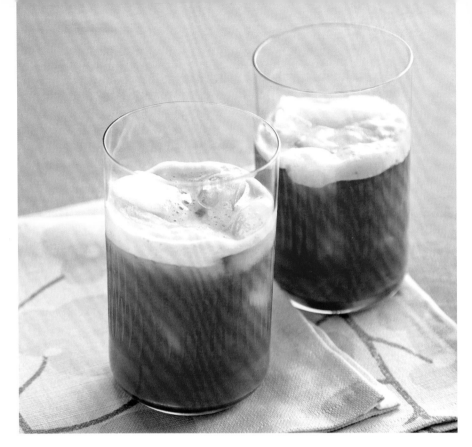

# 263

## red cabbage, grape + ginger
juice

SERVES 1

**100 g (3½ oz) red cabbage**

**1 apple**

**1 celery stick**

**2-cm (¾-inch) piece fresh root
ginger**

**12 red seedless grapes**

**ice cubes**

Trim the cabbage. Remove the stalk from the apple. Peel away any stringy bits from the celery. Peel the ginger.

Juice the prepared ingredients with the grapes.

Pour the juice over ice cubes in a glass and serve immediately.

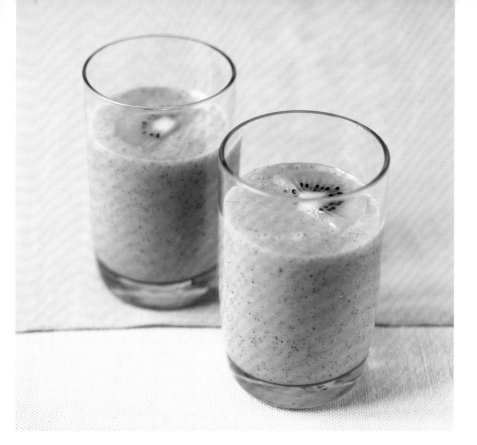

# 264

## kiwifruit + lime smoothie

SERVES 1

**3 kiwifruits, plus an extra
peeled slice to decorate**

**½ banana**

**50 g (1¾ oz) natural yogurt**

**1 teaspoon freshly squeezed
lime juice**

**drizzle of clear honey
(optional)**

**3-4 ice cubes**

Peel the kiwifruits, then roughly chop the flesh. Peel and roughly chop the banana.

Put the kiwifruits and banana in a blender or smoothie maker, add all the remaining ingredients and blend until smooth.

Pour the smoothie into a glass, decorate with a peeled kiwifruit slice and serve immediately.

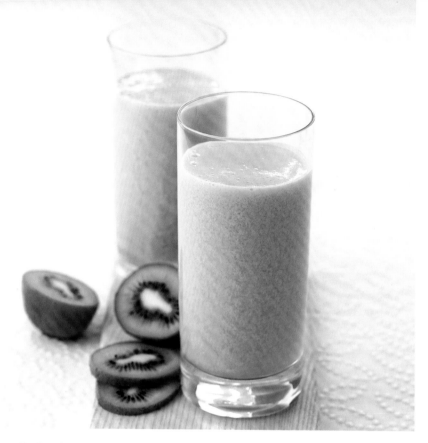

## 265

### pear, kiwifruit + lime juice

SERVES 1

**3 kiwifruits, plus extra slices to decorate (optional)**

**2 pears**

**½ lime**

**2–3 ice cubes (optional)**

Peel the kiwifruits. Remove the stalks from the pears.

Juice the kiwifruits and pears with the unpeeled lime half.

Pour the juice into a glass, then add a couple of ice cubes, if using, decorate with kiwifruit slices, if liked, and serve immediately.

## 266

### next time...

Swap the pears and lime for 300 g (10½ oz) green grapes.

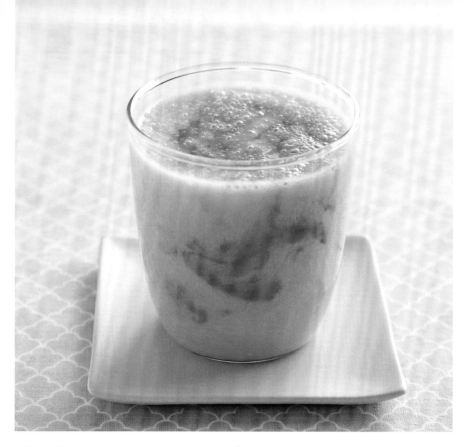

# 267

## strawberry + mango
### smoothie

SERVES 1

**1 orange**
**1 mango**
**60 g (2¼ oz) strawberries**
**100 ml (3½ fl oz) milk**
**1 tablespoon water**

Peel the orange. Peel and stone the mango, then roughly chop the flesh. Hull the strawberries.

Juice the orange. Transfer the orange juice to a blender or smoothie maker, add the mango and milk and blend until smooth. Pour the smoothie into a glass.

Blend the strawberries with the measured water until smooth, then pour into the glass on top of the mango mixture. Stir a little to create swirls of the strawberry mixture in the smoothie and serve immediately.

# 268

## banana + berry almond milk smoothie

SERVES 1

¼ large banana

200 g (7 oz) berries (such as strawberries, blueberries and raspberries), plus extra to decorate

75 ml (2½ fl oz) almond milk

1–2 ice cubes

Peel and roughly chop the banana. Put in a blender or smoothie maker, add the remaining ingredients and blend until smooth.

Pour the smoothie into a glass, decorate with a few berries and serve immediately.

# 269

## carrot + kiwifruit juice

SERVES 1

200 g (7 oz) carrots

1 kiwifruit, plus extra slices to decorate

ice cubes

Take the tops off the carrots and scrub. Peel the kiwifruit. Juice together.

Pour the juice into a glass over ice cubes, decorate with slices of kiwifruit and serve immediately.

# 270

## peanut butter, cocoa + banana smoothie

SERVES 1

1 banana

15 g (½ oz) peanut butter

15g (½ oz) chocolate or vanilla protein powder

1 teaspoon cocoa powder, plus extra to decorate

200 ml (7 fl oz) skimmed or semi-skimmed milk

few ice cubes (optional)

Peel the banana, then roughly chop. Put in a blender or smoothie maker, add all the remaining ingredients and blend until smooth.

Pour the smoothie into a glass, sprinkle over a little cocoa powder and serve immediately.

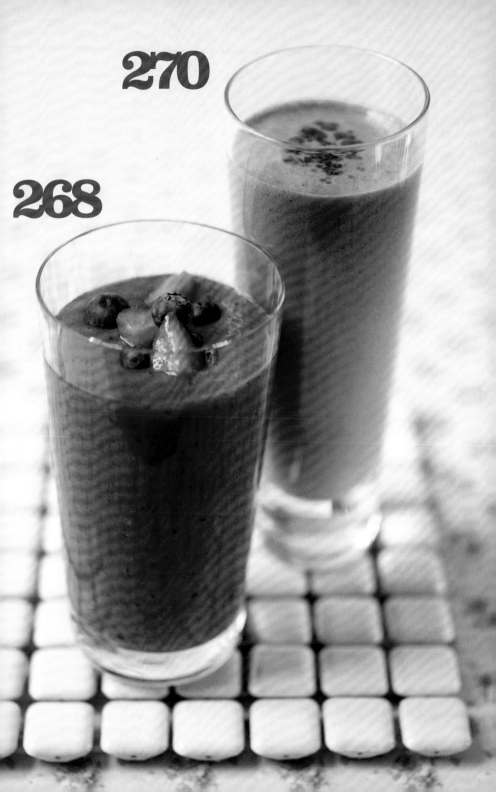

270

268

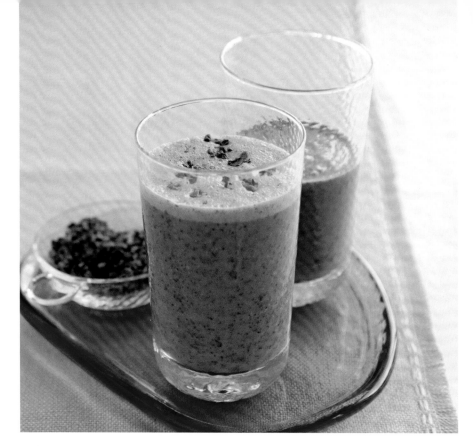

# 271

### cherry + chocolate smoothie

SERVES 2

**200 g (7 oz) cherries**

**100 g (3½ oz) blueberries**

**1 tablespoon cocoa nibs, plus extra to decorate**

**300 ml (10 fl oz) milk**

Stone the cherries. Juice the blueberries.

Transfer the blueberry juice to a blender or smoothie maker, add the cherries, cocoa nibs and milk and blend until smooth.

Pour the smoothie into glasses, decorate with some extra cocoa nibs and serve immediately.

# 272
## next time...

Fancy something more substantial? Add 1 tablespoon cashew nuts and 1 tablespoon rolled oats to the blender or smoothie maker with the other ingredients.

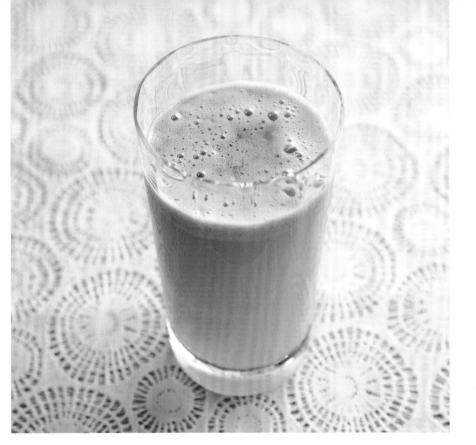

## 273

### grapefruit, kiwifruit + cucumber juice

SERVES 1

**2 grapefruits**

**1 kiwifruit**

**½ cucumber**

**1 apple, plus an extra slice to decorate (optional)**

Peel the grapefruits and kiwifruit. Trim the cucumber. Remove the stalk from the apple.

Juice all the ingredients together.

Pour the juice into a glass, decorate with an apple slice, if liked, and serve immediately.

## 274

### next time...

To spice this juice up, add a 2-cm (¾-inch) piece fresh root ginger, peeled and roughly chopped, to the other ingredients.

# 275

## gingered brussels sprout, carrot + apple
juice

SERVES 1

**1 carrot**

**1 apple**

**2-cm (¾-inch) piece fresh root ginger**

**6 Brussels sprouts**

Take the top off the carrot and then scrub. Remove the stalk from the apple. Peel the ginger.

Juice all the ingredients together.

Pour the juice into a glass and serve immediately.

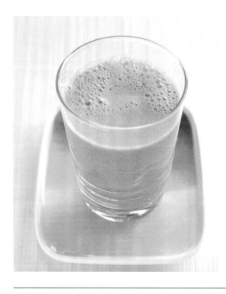

# 276

## carrot, ginger + radish
juice

SERVES 1

**100 g (3½ oz) carrots**

**100 g (3½ oz) radishes**

**2.5 cm (1 inch) fresh root ginger**

**ice cubes**

Take the tops off the carrots and then scrub. Trim the radishes. Peel the ginger.

Juice the carrots, radishes and ginger together.

Transfer the juice to a blender or food processor, add a couple of ice cubes and blend briefly.

Pour the juice over ice cubes in a glass and serve immediately.

## tip

This is a good juice if you have a cold or blocked sinuses.

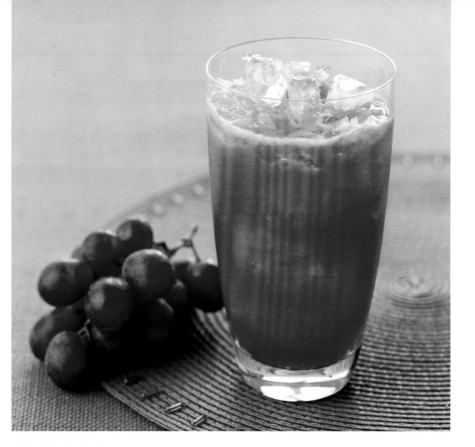

# 277

## grape + plum juice

SERVES 1

**300 g (10½ oz) plums, plus extra slices to decorate (optional)**

**150 g (5½ oz) red seedless grapes, plus extra to decorate (optional)**

**2–3 ice cubes, crushed**

Halve and stone the plums.

Juice the plums and grapes together.

Pour the juice into a glass, add the crushed ice cubes, decorate with grapes or plum slices, if liked, and serve immediately.

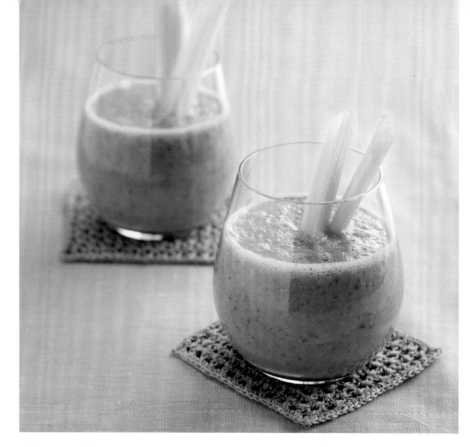

# 278

## herby spinach, celery + avocado smoothie

**SERVES 2**

**1 avocado**

**2 celery sticks, plus extra sticks to decorate**

**1 lime**

**1 garlic clove**

**30 g (1 oz) spinach**

**25 g (1 oz) parsley**

**1 teaspoon green powder (such as spirulina, wheatgrass or chlorella)**

**sea salt and freshly ground black pepper**

Peel and stone the avocado. Peel away the stringy bits from the celery. Peel the lime and garlic clove. Rinse the spinach.

Juice the lime and spinach together.

Transfer the juice to a blender or smoothie maker, add all the remaining ingredients except the seasoning and enough water to just cover and blend until smooth.

Season to taste with sea salt and black pepper and blend again briefly.

Pour the smoothie into glasses, add extra celery sticks to each glass and serve immediately.

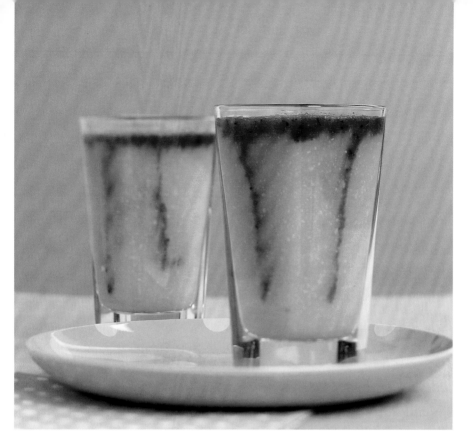

## 279

**mango, apple + blackcurrant**
smoothie

SERVES 1

**3 mangoes**

**200 g (7 oz) blackcurrants**

**100 ml (3½ fl oz) fresh apple juice**

Peel and stone the mangoes, then roughly chop the flesh. Remove the stalks from the blackcurrants.

Put the mangoes in a blender or smoothie maker, add the blackcurrants and apple juice and blend until smooth. Pour into a glass and serve immediately.

## 280
### next time...

Add 200 g (7 oz) blueberries to a blender or smoothie maker with 100 ml (3½ fl oz) apple juice, 300 ml (10 fl oz) natural yogurt and 2 tablespoons clear honey. Process until blended.

# 281

## beetroot, red cabbage + pineapple juice

SERVES 1

**2 beetroots**

**100 g (3½ oz) red cabbage**

**100 g (3½ oz) pineapple, plus an extra wedge to decorate**

**1 orange**

Trim the beetroot and then scrub or peel. Trim the cabbage. Cut the skin off the pineapple and remove the core if very tough. Peel the orange.

Juice all the ingredients together.

Pour the juice into a glass, decorate with a pineapple wedge and serve immediately.

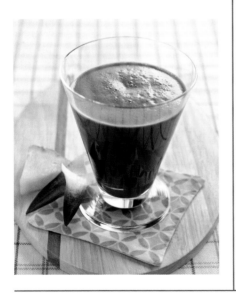

# 282

## simple mango smoothie

SERVES 1

**½ large mango**

**100 g (3½ oz) natural yogurt**

**100 ml (3½ fl oz) water**

Peel and stone the mango, then roughly chop the flesh.

Put the mango in a blender or smoothie maker, add the yogurt and measured water and blend until smooth.

Pour the smoothie into a glass and serve immediately.

### tip

Yellow-fleshed mango is high in beta-carotene, important in helping to guard against some cancers.

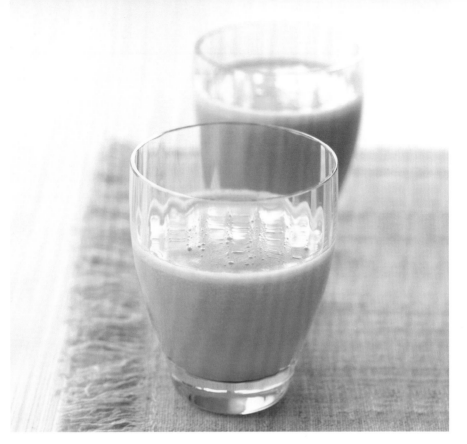

# 283

## pear, grapefruit + celery
juice

SERVES 1

**75 g (2¾ oz) grapefruit**
**125 g (4½ oz) lettuce**
**75 g (2¾ oz) celery**
**50 g (1¾ oz) pear**
**ice cubes (optional)**

Peel the grapefruit. Separate the lettuce leaves. Peel away any stringy bits from the celery. Remove the stalk from the pear.

Juice all the prepared ingredients together.

Pour the juice over ice cubes, if using, in a glass and serve immediately.

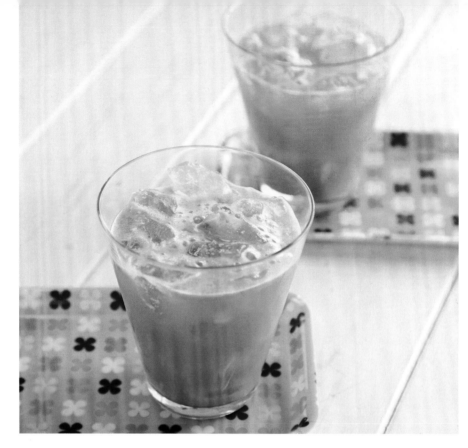

# 284

## summer salad juice

**SERVES 1**

**2 little gem lettuces**

**2 carrots**

**1 apple**

**1 celery stick**

**¼ cucumber**

**2 salad tomatoes**

**ice cubes**

Separate the lettuce leaves. Take the tops off the carrots and then scrub. Remove the stalk from the apple. Peel away any stringy bits from the celery.

Juice the prepared ingredients with the cucumber and tomatoes.

Pour the juice over ice cubes in a glass and serve immediately.

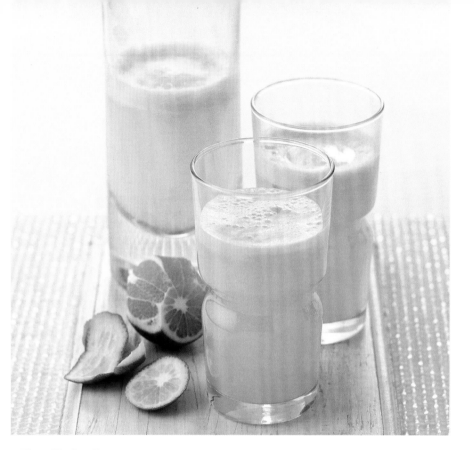

# 285

## grapefruit + orange juice

**1 large orange**

**½ grapefruit**

**1 lime**

**ice cubes or sparkling
mineral water**

Peel all the citrus fruits. If you like, reserve some of the lime rind to decorate.

Juice all the fruits together.

Pour the juice over ice cubes in a glass or, if you want a longer drink, dilute it with an equal amount of sparkling mineral water. Decorate with curls of lime rind, if liked, and serve immediately.

## 286

# kiwifruit, mango + raspberry smoothie

SERVES 2

**3 kiwifruits**

**150 g (5½ oz) lemon or orange yogurt**

**1 small mango**

**2 tablespoons fresh orange or apple juice**

**150 g (5½ oz) raspberries**

**1–2 teaspoons clear honey**

Peel and roughly chop the kiwifruits. Put in a blender or smoothie maker and blend to a purée.

Spoon the kiwifruit purée into glasses and top each with a spoonful of the yogurt, spreading the yogurt to the sides of the glasses.

Peel and stone the mango, then roughly chop the flesh.

Blend the mango with the orange or apple juice to a purée. Spoon the mango purée on top of the kiwifruit purée and yogurt, then top with another layer of yogurt.

Blend the raspberries to a purée, then press through a sieve over a bowl to extract the seeds. Check the raspberry purée for sweetness and add honey to taste, then spoon into the glasses. Serve immediately.

## 287

# spicy pear + parsnip juice

SERVES 1

**1 large pear, preferably red**

**125 g (4½ oz) parsnip**

**15 g (½ oz) fresh root ginger**

**125 ml (4 fl oz) sparkling mineral water**

Cut several long, thin slices from the pear and reserve. Peel the parsnip and ginger.

Juice the parsnip and ginger together, then the pear.

Pour the juice over the reserved pear slices in a glass, top up with the sparkling mineral water and serve immediately.

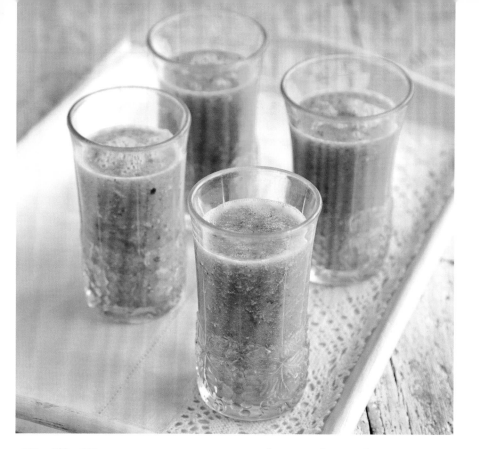

# 288

## watermelon, mint + berry
smoothie

SERVES 4

**1 kg (2 lb 4 oz) watermelon**
**14–16 strawberries**
**12 mint leaves**
**small handful of ice cubes**

Peel the melon as close to the skin as possible and deseed, then roughly chop the flesh. Hull the strawberries.

Place all the ingredients in a blender or smoothie maker and blend until smooth.

Pour into glasses and serve immediately.

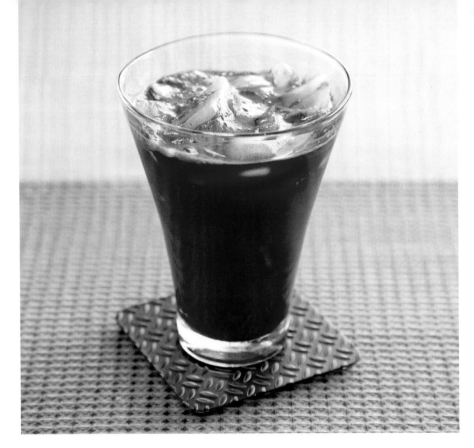

# 289

## red pepper, beetroot + watercress juice

SERVES 1

**1 red pepper**

**1 beetroot**

**2 carrots**

**½ lemon**

**50 g (1¾ oz) watercress**

**ice cubes**

**coarsely ground black pepper, to decorate (optional)**

Core and deseed the red pepper. Trim the beetroot and then scrub or peel. Take the tops off the carrots and then scrub. Peel the lemon half.

Juice the red pepper, beetroot, carrots, lemon and watercress together.

Pour the juice over ice cubes in a glass, sprinkle with black pepper, if liked, and serve immediately.

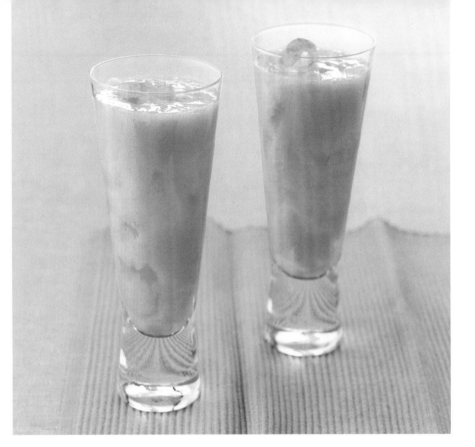

# 290

## apricot + pineapple juice

SERVES 1

**70 g (2½ oz) ready-to-eat dried apricots**

**350 ml (12 fl oz) pineapple juice**

**2–3 ice cubes**

Roughly chop the dried apricots and put them in a large bowl. Pour over the pineapple juice, cover and leave to stand overnight in the refrigerator.

Transfer the apricots and juice to a blender or smoothie maker and blend until thick and smooth.

Pour the juice into a glass, add the ice cubes and serve immediately.

# 291

## red pepper, cucumber + broccoli juice

SERVES 1

**2 red peppers**

**½ cucumber**

**100 g (3½ oz) broccoli**

**1 lime, plus extra slices to decorate**

**ice cubes**

Core and deseed the red peppers. Trim the cucumber and broccoli. Peel the lime.

Juice all the prepared ingredients together.

Pour the juice over ice cubes in a glass, decorate with lime slices and serve immediately.

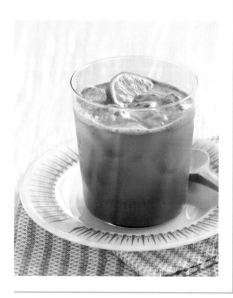

# 292

## gazpacho mix

SERVES 1

**½ red pepper**

**¼ cucumber**

**1 small garlic clove**

**2 salad tomatoes**

**1 celery stick**

**small handful of mixed parsley and basil leaves**

**ice cubes**

Core and deseed the red pepper, then roughly chop. Peel the cucumber. Peel the garlic.

Put all the ingredients in a blender or food processor and blend together – you can leave the mixture a little chunky if you like.

Pour the mixture over ice cubes in a glass or a bowl and serve immediately.

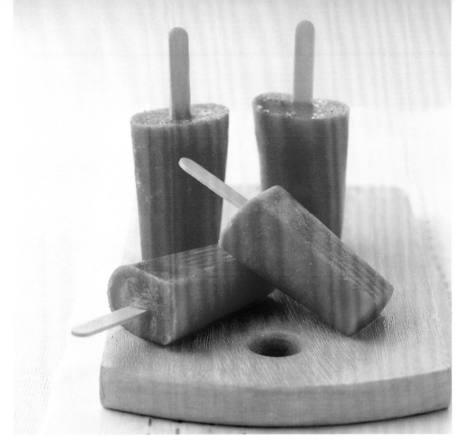

# 293

## strawberry, mango + orange
lollies

MAKES ABOUT 4–5 LOLLIES

**125 g (4½ oz) strawberries**

**1 small mango**

**300 ml (10 fl oz) fresh orange juice**

Hull the strawberries, then put them in a freezerproof container and freeze for 2 hours or overnight.

Peel and stone the mango, then roughly chop the flesh.

Put the mango, frozen strawberries and orange juice in a blender or food smoothie maker and blend until smooth.

Pour the mixture into 4–5 lolly moulds and freeze until set before serving.

## 295

### tomato + asparagus juice

SERVES 1

**1 carrot**

**100 g (3½ oz) asparagus spears**

**100 g (3½ oz) sweet tomatoes**

**dash of Worcestershire sauce, to taste**

Take the top off the carrot and then scrub.

Juice the carrot, asparagus and tomatoes together, then add the Worcestershire sauce to taste.

Pour the juice into a glass and serve immediately.

## 294

### cranberry, cucumber + orange juice

SERVES 1

**1 orange**

**50 g (1¾ oz) cucumber**

**100 ml (3½ fl oz) cranberry juice**

**ice cubes**

Peel the orange and trim the cucumber.

Juice the orange and cucumber together, then mix with the cranberry juice.

Pour the combined juices into a glass over ice and serve immediately.

## 296

### next time...

Swap the asparagus spears for 100 g (3½ oz) fine green beans, trimmed.

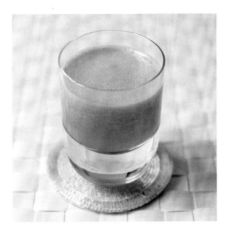

## 297

## pineapple, green bean + courgette juice

SERVES 1

½ pineapple
½ courgette
10 fine green beans
½ lime

Cut the skin off the pineapple and remove the core if very tough, then roughly chop the flesh. Trim the courgette and beans.

Juice the prepared ingredients with the unpeeled lime half.

Pour the juice into a glass and serve immediately.

There is no need to remove the core of the pineapple unless it is very hard.

## 298

## fennel, orange + flax seed juice

SERVES 1

1 orange
1 fennel bulb
1 carrot
½ teaspoon ground flax seeds

Peel the orange. Trim the fennel. Take the top off the carrot and then scrub.

Juice the orange, fennel and carrot together, then stir the ground flax seeds into the juice.

Pour the juice into a glass and serve immediately.

Fennel helps to digest fats, which will give support to your liver.

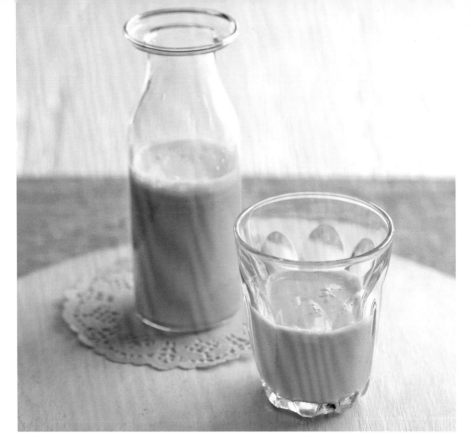

## 299

**pomegranate, carrot + radish**
juice

SERVES 1

**1 pomegranate**
**1 apple**
**1 orange**
**2 carrots**
**25 g (1 oz) radish sprouts**

Remove the seeds from the pomegranate by cutting the fruit in half, then holding the halved fruit over a bowl and hitting the skin with a wooden spoon so that the seeds fall into the bowl.

Remove the stalk from the apple. Peel the orange. Juice all the ingredients together.

Pour the juice into a glass and serve immediately.

## 300
### next time...

To spice this juice up, replace the pomegranate seeds with ½ red chilli and a pinch of freshly ground black pepper.

# 301

## carrot, spinach + spirulina juice

SERVES 1

**250 g (9 oz) carrots**
**250 g (9 oz) spinach**
**25 g (1 oz) parsley**
**1 teaspoon spirulina powder**

Take the tops off the carrots and then scrub. Rinse the spinach.

Juice the carrots and spinach with the parsley, then stir in the spirulina.

Pour the juice into a glass and serve immediately.

Spirulina is a freshwater algae supplement and a great energy booster.

# 302

## fennel, apple + carrot juice

SERVES 1

**1 fennel bulb**
**1 apple**
**1 carrot**
**pinch of grated nutmeg, to decorate**

Trim the fennel. Remove the stalk from the apple. Take the top off the carrot and then scrub.

Juice all the ingredients together. Pour the juice into a glass, sprinkle with the nutmeg and serve immediately.

Fennel is a natural diuretic.

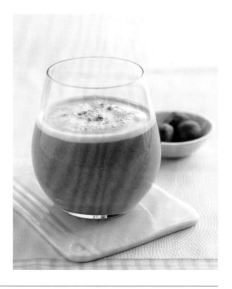

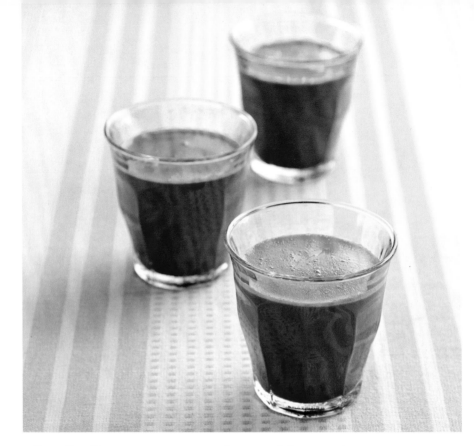

# 303

## spring cabbage, beetroot + orange juice

SERVES 1

**175 g (6 oz) spring cabbage**

**1 beetroot**

**1 orange**

Trim the cabbage. Trim the beetroot and then scrub or peel. Peel the orange.

Juice all the ingredients together.

Pour the juice into a glass and serve immediately.

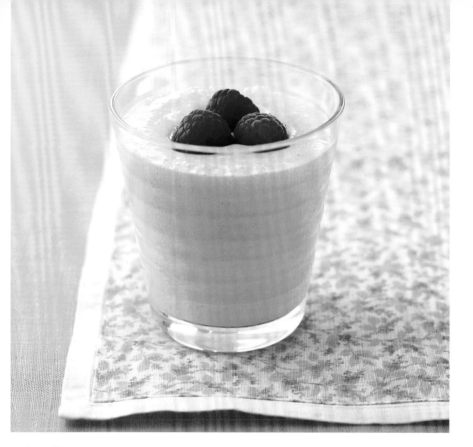

# 304

## **peach** smoothie

SERVES 1

**1 large peach**
**150 g (5½ oz) natural yogurt**
**50 ml (2 fl oz) milk**
**raspberries, to decorate**

Peel, halve and stone the peach, then roughly chop the flesh.

Put the peach in a blender or smoothie maker, add the yogurt and milk and blend until smooth.

Pour the smoothie into a glass, decorate with raspberries and serve immediately.

# 305

## sweet potato + spinach
juice

SERVES 1

**1 large carrot**

**2 celery sticks**

**1 sweet potato**

**60 g (2¼ oz) spinach**

Take the top off the carrot and then scrub. Peel away any stringy bits from the celery. Peel the sweet potato. Rinse the spinach.

Juice all the ingredients together.

Pour the juice into a glass and serve immediately.

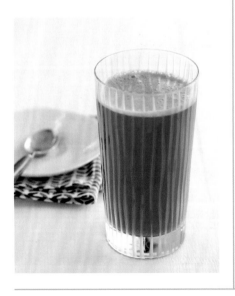

# 306

## raspberry, cranberry + pomegranate juice

SERVES 1

**1 apple**

**2-cm (¾-inch) piece fresh root ginger**

**25 g (1 oz) fresh or frozen (defrosted) cranberries**

**50 g (1¾ oz) pomegranate seeds**

**100 g (3½ oz) raspberries**

**large pinch of grated nutmeg**

Remove the stalk from the apple. Peel the ginger.

Juice all the fruits with the ginger.

Pour the juice into a glass, stir in the grated nutmeg and serve immediately.

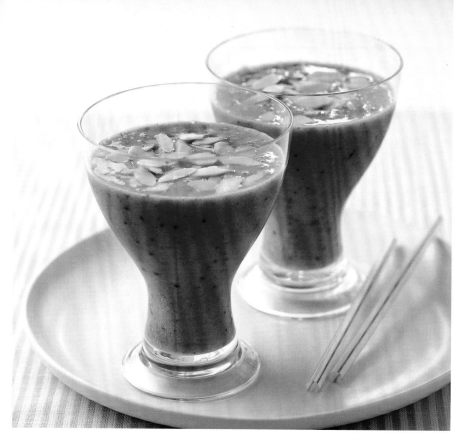

# 307

## strawberry + soya smoothie

**SERVES 1**

**100 g (3½ oz) fresh or frozen
strawberries**

**2 kiwifruits**

**200 ml (7 fl oz) soya milk**

**ice cubes (optional)**

**25 g (1 oz) flaked almonds,
to decorate (optional)**

Hull the strawberries if using fresh. Peel the kiwifruits.

Put the fruits into a blender or smoothie maker, add the soya milk and blend briefly. If you are using fresh rather than frozen strawberries, add a few ice cubes and blend until smooth.

Pour the smoothie into a glass, decorate with flaked almonds, if liked, and serve immediately.

## 308

# kiwifruit, apple + **ginger** sparkler

SERVES 1

**3 kiwifruits**

**2-cm (¾-inch) piece fresh root ginger**

**1 apple**

**ice cubes (optional)**

**300 ml (10 fl oz) sparkling mineral water**

Peel the kiwifruits and ginger. Remove the stalk from the apple.

Juice the kiwifruits, ginger and apple together.

Pour the juice over ice cubes, if using, in a glass, top up with the measured mineral water and serve immediately.

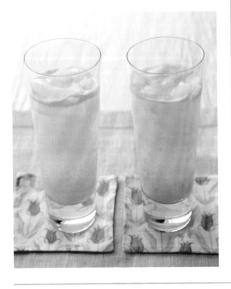

## 309

# feverfew infusion

SERVES 1

**4 large feverfew sprigs**

**3–4 fresh or dried hibiscus flowers**

**pared strip of lemon rind**

**200 ml (7 fl oz) boiling water**

**1 teaspoon freshly squeezed lemon juice**

**clear honey, to taste**

Put 3 of the feverfew sprigs, the hibiscus and lemon rind in a cup and pour over the measured boiling water. Leave to infuse for 4–5 minutes.

Lift out the hibiscus, feverfew and lemon rind and stir in the lemon juice and a little honey, to taste. Decorate with the remaining feverfew sprig and serve hot.

### tip

Feverfew is renowned as a cure for headaches and fever because of its ability to improve blood vessel functioning and reduce inflammation. Both the flowers and leaves of the herb can be used.

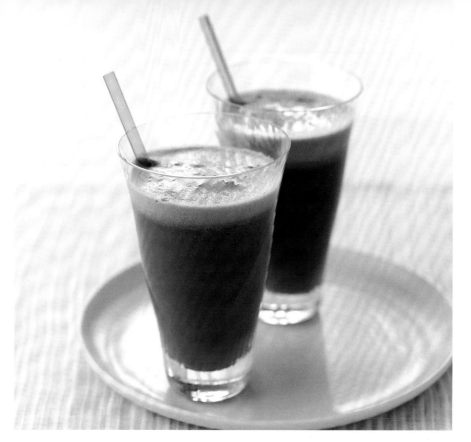

# 310

## prune, pear + spinach
juice

SERVES 1

**250 g (9 oz) pears, plus extra
slices to decorate (optional)**

**125 g (4½ oz) spinach**

**25 g (1 oz) pitted prunes**

**ice cubes (optional)**

Remove the stalks from the pears. Rinse the spinach.

Juice the pears, spinach and prunes together.

Pour the juice over ice cubes, if using, in a glass, decorate with pear slices, if liked, and serve immediately.

This juice is rich in fibre, with good cleansing properties to stimulate the abdomen and improve your digestion.

**197**

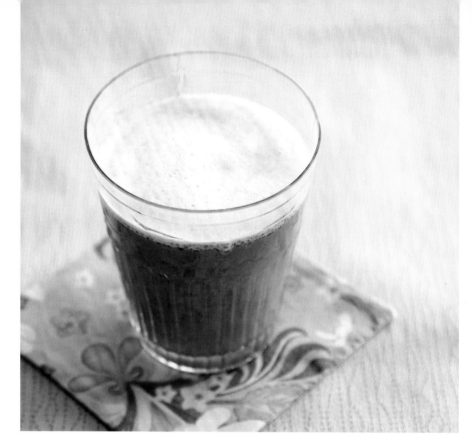

# 311

## broccoli, apple + coriander
juice

SERVES 1

**150 g (5½ oz) broccoli**

**2 celery sticks**

**2 apples**

**10 g (¼ oz) coriander leaves**

**1–2 teaspoons avocado oil**

Trim the broccoli. Peel away any stringy bits from the celery. Remove the stalks from the apples.

Juice the broccoli with the celery, apple and coriander, then stir in the avocado oil.

Pour the juice into a glass and serve immediately.

# 312
## next time...

Juice ¼ head broccoli, trimmed, with 2 celery sticks, any stringy bits removed, 200 g (7oz) peeled and deseeded watermelon chunks and ½ cucumber, trimmed. Serve immediately over ice cubes.

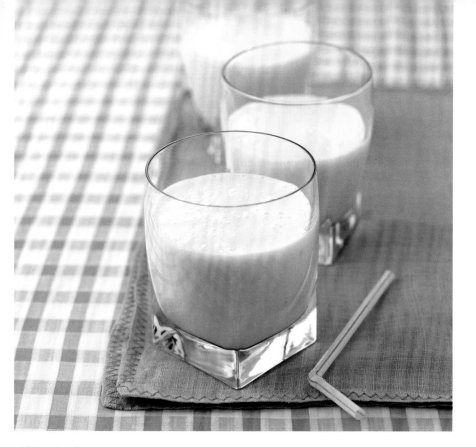

# 313

## mango + orange smoothie

SERVES 1

**1 mango**

**200 ml (7 fl oz) fresh orange juice**

**150 ml (5 fl oz) semi-skimmed milk**

**3 tablespoons fromage frais**

**2–3 ice cubes**

Peel the banana, then roughly chop. Peel and stone the mango, then roughly chop the flesh.

Put all the ingredients in a blender or smoothie maker and blend until smooth.

Pour the smoothie into glasses and serve immediately.

# 314

## mixed currants + apple juice

SERVES 1

**2 apples**

**300 g (10½ oz) blackcurrants**

**100 g (3½ oz) redcurrants**

**blackcurrant or redcurrant sprig, to decorate**

Remove the stalks from the apples and the currants.

Juice the apples and currants together.

Pour the juice into a glass, decorate with a blackcurrant or redcurrant sprig and serve immediately.

# 315

## nectarine, orange + **raspberry** smoothie

SERVES 1

**1 nectarine**

**1 orange**

**150 g (5½ oz) raspberries**

Halve and stone the nectarine. Peel and segment the orange.

Put all the fruits in a blender or smoothie maker and blend until smooth.

Pour into a glass and serve immediately.

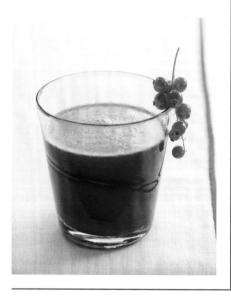

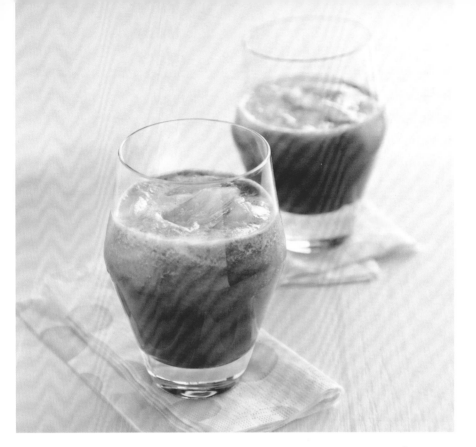

# 316

## clementine, cherry + apricot
juice

SERVES 1

**2 clementines**

**6 cherries**

**1 apricot**

**1 apple**

**6 red seedless grapes**

**1 lemon grass stalk**

**ice cubes**

Peel the clementines. Stone the cherries. Halve and stone the apricot. Remove the stalk from the apple.

Juice the prepared ingredients with the grapes and lemon grass.

Pour the juice over ice cubes in a glass and serve immediately.

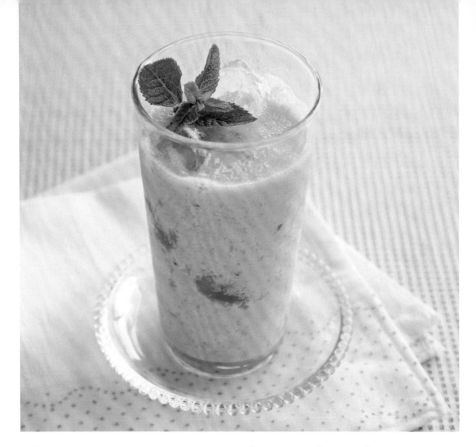

# 317

## gooseberry, almond + elderflower smoothie

**SERVES 1**

**125 g (4½ oz) gooseberries**

**½ lime**

**small handful of mint, plus an extra sprig to decorate**

**30 g (1 oz) ground almonds**

**150 ml (5 fl oz) non-dairy milk**

**1 teaspoon elderflower cordial**

Snip off the tip and flower end of the gooseberries. Peel the lime half. Pull the mint leaves off their stalks.

Juice the lime with the mint.

Transfer the juice to a blender or smoothie maker, add all the remaining ingredients and blend until smooth.

Pour the smoothie into a glass, decorate with a mint sprig and serve immediately.

# 318

## beetroot + chlorella
juice

SERVES 1

**1 beetroot**

**1 apple**

**½ cucumber**

**40 g (1½ oz) kale**

**2-cm (¾-inch) piece fresh root ginger**

**½ teaspoon chlorella powder**

**ice cubes**

Trim the beetroot and then scrub or peel. Remove the stalk from the apple. Trim the cucumber. Cut any really woody stalks off the kale. Peel the ginger.

Juice the kale with the beetroot, apple, cucumber and ginger, then stir in the chlorella powder.

Pour the juice over ice cubes in a glass and serve immediately.

**tip**

Chlorella is an oriental algae that is packed with protein – twice as much as spinach.

# 319

## banana + chocolate
smoothie

SERVES 2

**1 banana**

**2 tablespoons organic cocoa powder, plus extra to decorate**

**300 ml (10 fl oz) semi-skimmed milk**

**100 ml (3½ fl oz) fresh apple juice**

**2 large scoops vanilla ice cream**

Peel the banana, then roughly chop. Put in a blender or smoothie maker, add the cocoa powder, milk, apple juice and ice cream and blend until smooth.

Pour the mixture into glasses, sprinkle with cocoa powder and serve immediately.

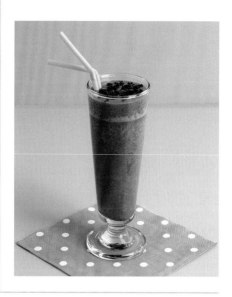

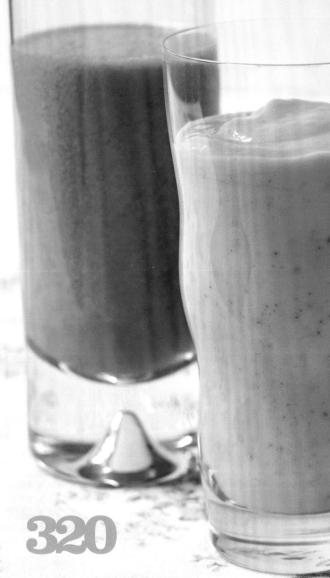

321

320

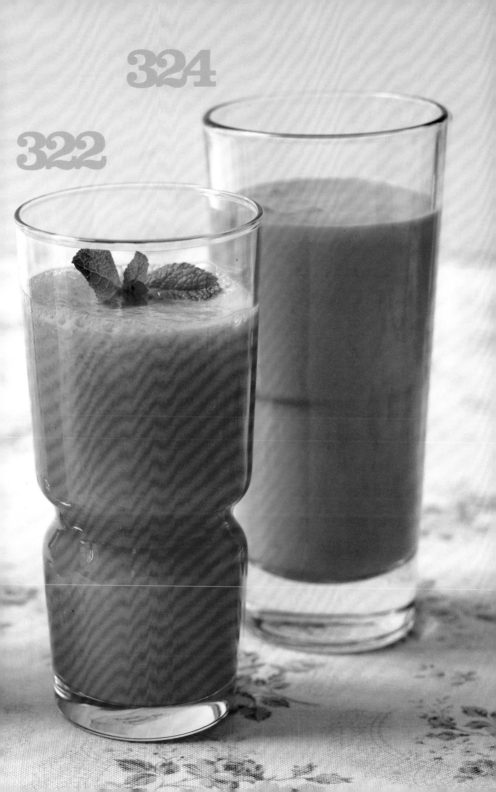

322

324

# 320

## apple, carrot + banana
## smoothie

SERVES 1

**2 apples**

**1 carrot**

**1 banana**

**2 ice cubes (optional)**

Remove the stalks from the apples. Take the top off the carrot and then scrub. Peel the banana, then roughly chop.

Juice the apples and carrot together.

Transfer the juice to a blender or smoothie maker, add the banana and ice cubes, if using, and blend until smooth.

Pour the smoothie into a glass and serve immediately.

# 321

## banana + avocado
## smoothie

SERVES 1

**1 banana**

**½ avocado**

**150 ml (5 fl oz) almond milk**

**drizzle of clear honey, to taste (optional)**

Peel and slice the banana, put it in a freezerproof container and freeze for at least 2 hours or overnight.

Peel and stone the avocado.

Transfer the frozen banana to a blender or smoothie maker and blend until smooth. Add the avocado and almond milk and blend again. Sweeten to taste with honey, if liked.

Pour the smoothie into a glass and serve immediately.

# 322

## orange, carrot + ginger
juice

SERVES 1

**2 carrots**

**2 oranges**

**2-cm (¾-inch) piece fresh root ginger**

**8 mint leaves, plus extra to decorate**

Take the tops off the carrots and then scrub. Peel the oranges and the ginger.

Juice all the ingredients together.

Pour the juice into a glass, decorate with extra mint leaves and serve immediately.

# 323

## next time...

Juice 2 carrots, tops trimmed and then scrubbed, with 2 sweet apples, stalks removed, 2-cm (¾-inch) piece fresh root ginger, peeled, and a few mint leaves.

# 324

## mango + spinach
smoothie

SERVES 1

**½ mango**

**25 g (1 oz) spinach**

**75 ml (2½ fl oz) skimmed milk**

**75 ml (2½ fl oz) freshly squeezed orange juice**

**10 g (¼ oz) raw cashew nuts**

**juice of 1 lime**

Peel and chop the mango. Rinse the spinach.

Put all the ingredients in a blender or smoothie maker and blend until smooth.

Pour the smoothie into a glass and serve immediately.

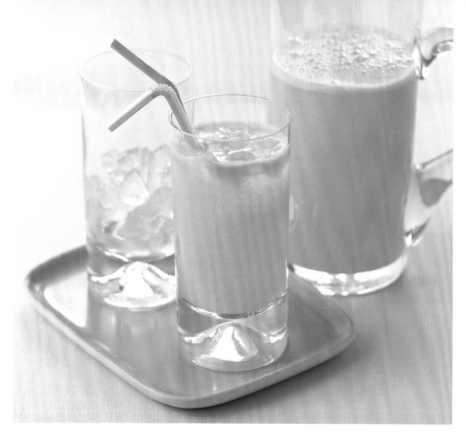

# 325

## orange + passionfruit
### sparkler

SERVES 1

**100 g (3½ oz) orange**

**1 passionfruit**

**100 ml (3½ fl oz) sparkling
mineral water**

**2–3 ice cubes**

Peel the orange and then juice.

Halve the passionfruit and scoop out the seeds
and pulp into a tea strainer set over a cup. Press
the pulp with the back of a teaspoon to extract the
juice.

Mix the orange juice with the passionfruit juice
and measured mineral water.

Pour the drink over the ice cubes in a glass and
serve immediately.

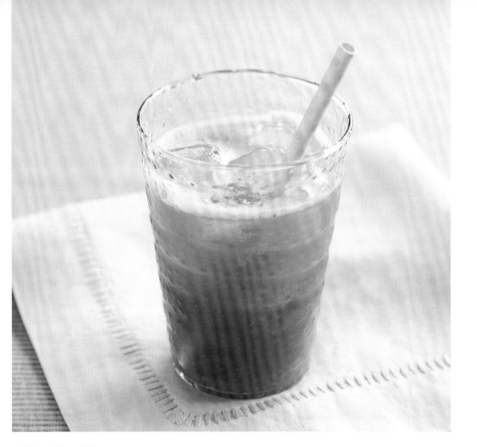

# 326

## gingered pear juice

**SERVES 1**

**5 pears**

**2-cm (¾-inch) piece fresh root ginger**

**large pinch of ground cinnamon**

**ice cubes**

Remove the stalks from the pears. Peel the ginger.

Juice the ginger with the pears, then stir in the cinnamon.

Pour the juice over ice cubes in a glass and serve immediately.

## 327

# mango + passionfruit
## smoothie

SERVES 4

**1 large mango**
**750 g (1 lb 10 oz) natural yogurt**
**1–2 tablespoons agave nectar, to taste**
**1 vanilla pod, split in half lengthways**
**4 passionfruits**

Peel and stone the mango, then roughly chop the flesh. Add the mango to a blender or smoothie maker and blend to a purée.

Add the yogurt and agave nectar, according to taste, to a large bowl, scrape in the seeds from the vanilla pod and beat together. Gently fold in the mango purée and spoon into glasses.

Halve the passionfruits, scoop out the seeds and pulp and spoon over the smoothie. Serve immediately.

## 328

# papaya + peach
## smoothie

SERVES 1

**¼ large papaya**
**1 large peach**
**100 ml (3½ fl oz) grapefruit juice**

Peel and deseed the papaya, then roughly chop the flesh. Halve and stone the peach.

Put the papaya and peach in a blender or smoothie maker, add the grapefruit juice and blend until smooth.

Pour the smoothie into a glass and serve immediately.

## 329

## next time...

Swap the papaya for ¾ cantaloupe melon, peeled as close to the skin as possible and deseeded, and the grapefruit juice for orange juice.

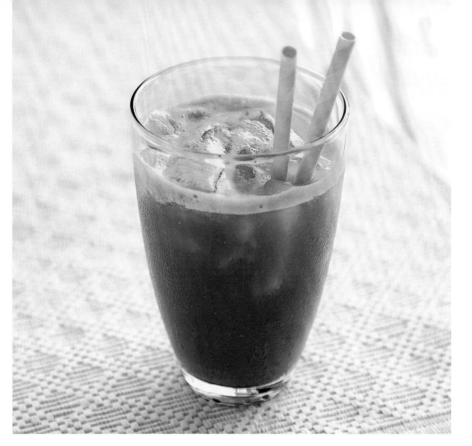

# 330

## tropical green juice

SERVES 1

**180 g (6¼ oz) pineapple**

**1 apple**

**50 g (1¾ oz) kale**

**20 g (¾ oz) spinach**

**1 teaspoon green powder
(such as wheatgrass,
spirulina or chlorella)**

**ice cubes**

Cut the skin off the pineapple and remove the core if very tough. Remove the stalk from the apple. Cut any really woody stalks off the kale. Rinse the spinach.

Juice the prepared ingredients together, then stir in the green powder.

Pour the juice over ice cubes in a glass and serve immediately.

# 331

## papaya, orange + strawberry juice

SERVES 1

**¼ large papaya, plus an extra wedge, to decorate**

**2 oranges**

**125 g (4½ oz) strawberries**

Peel and deseed the papaya. Peel the oranges and hull the strawberries.

Juice all the fruits together. Pour the juice into a glass, decorate with a papaya wedge and serve immediately.

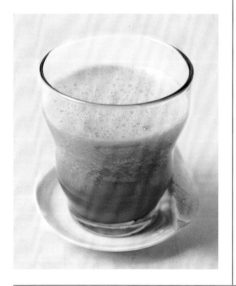

# 332

## goji + blueberry juice

SERVES 1

**30 g (1 oz) goji berries**

**150 g (5½ oz) blueberries**

**100 ml (3½ fl oz) pure pomegranate juice**

Soak the goji berries in water for at least an hour until they have plumped up.

Drain the berries, then transfer to a blender or smoothie maker, add the blueberries and pomegranate juice and blend until smooth.

Pour the juice into a glass and serve immediately.

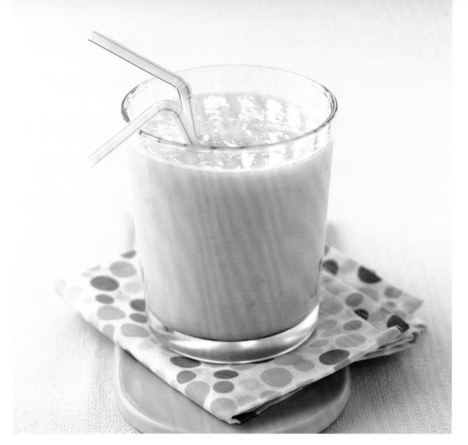

# 333

### banana + mango smoothie

SERVES 3

**1 large banana, plus extra slices to decorate (optional)**

**1 large mango**

**150 g (5½ oz) natural yogurt**

**300 ml (10 fl oz) pineapple juice**

Peel and slice the banana, then put in a freezerproof container and freeze for at least 2 hours or overnight.

Peel and stone the mango, then roughly chop the flesh.

Put the frozen banana, mango, yogurt and pineapple juice in a blender or smoothie maker and blend until smooth.

Pour the smoothie into glasses, decorate each with a banana slice, if liked, and serve immediately.

# 334

## citrus + wheatgrass
juice

SERVES 1

**1 lime**
**1 orange**
**1 grapefruit**
**1 teaspoon agave syrup**
**½ tablespoon wheatgrass powder**

Peel the citrus fruits, then juice them together.

Stir the agave syrup and wheatgrass powder into the juice.

Pour the juice into a glass and serve immediately.

# 335

## blueberry + almond
smoothie

SERVES 1

**½ banana**
**150 g (5½ oz) frozen blueberries**
**10 g (¼ oz) rolled oats**
**2 teaspoons almond butter**
**drop of vanilla extract**
**almond milk, as needed**

Peel the banana and roughly chop. Put in a blender or smoothie maker with the oats, almond butter and vanilla extract and then blend with as much almond milk as needed to achieve your desired consistency.

Pour the smoothie into a glass and serve immediately.

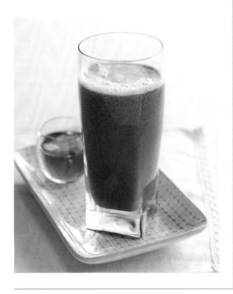

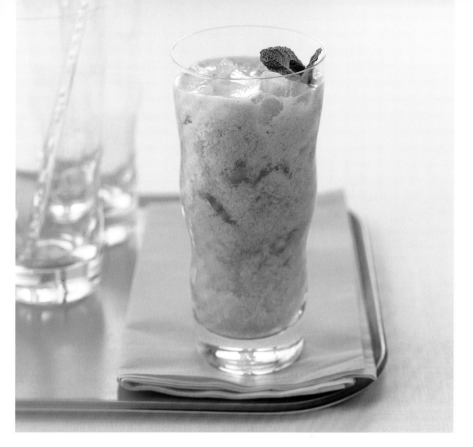

# 336

## peach + ginger juice

**SERVES 1**

**250 g (9 oz) peaches**

**2.5-cm (1-inch) piece fresh root ginger**

**ice cubes**

**splash of sparkling mineral water**

**2 mint leaves, to decorate**

Halve and stone the peaches. Peel the ginger.

Juice the peaches and ginger together.

Pour the juice over ice cubes in a tall glass and add the sparkling mineral water. Decorate with the mint leaves and serve immediately.

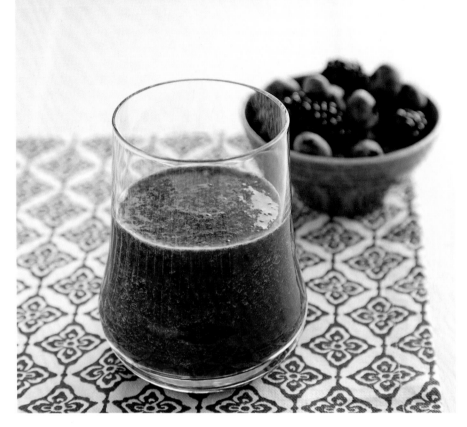

# 337

## blackberry, blueberry + apple juice

SERVES 1

**1 apple**

**200 g (7 oz) blackberries**

**100 g (3½ oz) blueberries**

Remove the stalk from the apple, then juice with the berries.

Pour the juice into a glass and serve immediately.

# 338

## strawberry, kiwifruit + banana smoothie

SERVES 1

250 g (9 oz) strawberries

1 kiwifruit

½ large banana

1 tablespoon spirulina powder

1 tablespoon flax seeds

2 ice cubes

Hull the strawberries. Peel the kiwifruit. Peel the banana, then roughly chop.

Juice the strawberries and kiwifruit together.

Transfer the juice to a blender or smoothie maker, add the banana, spirulina, flax seeds and ice cubes and blend until smooth.

Pour the smoothie into a glass and serve immediately.

**tip**

Spirulina is high in calcium, magnesium and vitamin A.

# 339

## blueberry, cranberry + pomegranate juice

SERVES 1

1 kiwifruit

1 carrot

25 g (1 oz) fresh or frozen (defrosted) cranberries

50 g (1¾ oz) pomegranate seeds

100 g (3½ oz) blueberries

Peel the kiwifruit. Take the top off the carrot and then scrub.

Juice all the ingredients together.

Pour the juice into a glass and serve immediately.

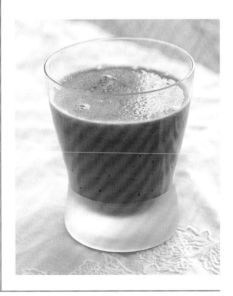

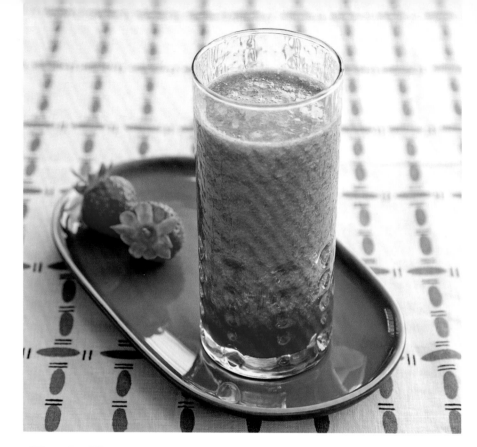

# 340

## berry, cabbage + grape
juice

SERVES 1

**12 strawberries, plus extra to decorate**

**100 g (3½ oz) green cabbage**

**100 g (3½ oz) blueberries**

**100 g (3½ oz) raspberries**

**8 seedless grapes**

Hull the strawberries and trim the cabbage.

Juice all the ingredients together.

Pour the juice into a glass, decorate with extra strawberries and serve immediately.

# 341
## next time...

Juice 250 g (9 oz) each of carrots, tops trimmed and then scrubbed, and cabbage, trimmed, then serve immediately over ice cubes. This quick juice soothes upset stomachs.

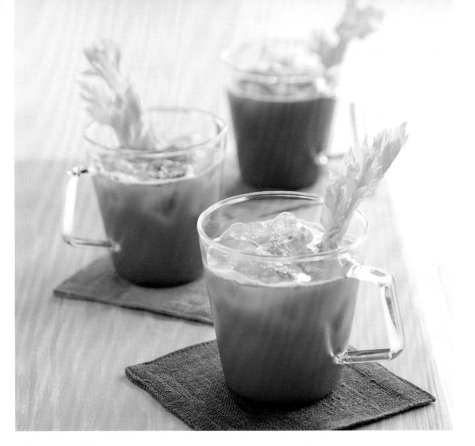

# 342

## cucumber, kale + wheatgrass
juice

SERVES 1

**1 apple**

**½ cucumber**

**2 celery sticks, plus an extra
trimmed stick to decorate**

**1 lemon**

**30 g (1 oz) kale**

**15 g (½ oz) parsley**

**1 teaspoon wheatgrass
powder**

**ice cubes**

Remove the stalk from the apple. Trim the cucumber.
Peel away any stringy bits from the celery. Peel the
lemon. Cut any really woody stalks off the kale.

Juice the prepared ingredients with the parsley,
then whisk in the wheatgrass powder.

Pour the juice over ice cubes in a glass, add a
trimmed celery stick and serve immediately.

# 343

## minty apple tea

SERVES 2

**3 apples**

**large handful of mint, plus extra sprigs
to decorate**

**200 ml (7 fl oz) mint tea, chilled**

**ice cubes**

Remove the stalks from the apples and
pull the mint leaves off their stalks.

Juice the apples and mint together,
then stir in the chilled mint tea.

Pour the drink over ice cubes in
glasses, decorate each glass with a
mint sprig and serve immediately.

# 344

## minty carrot + apple juice

SERVES 1

**4 large carrots**

**1 romaine lettuce**

**½ cucumber**

**large bunch of mint**

**⅔ small apple**

**ice cubes**

Take the tops off the carrots and then
scrub. Separate the lettuce leaves. Trim
the cucumber. Pull the mint leaves off
their stalks. Remove the stalk from the
apple.

Juice all the prepared ingredients
together.

Pour the juice over ice cubes in a glass
and serve immediately.

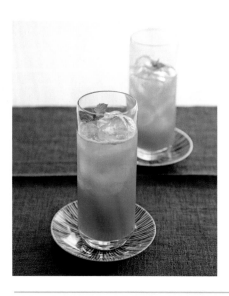

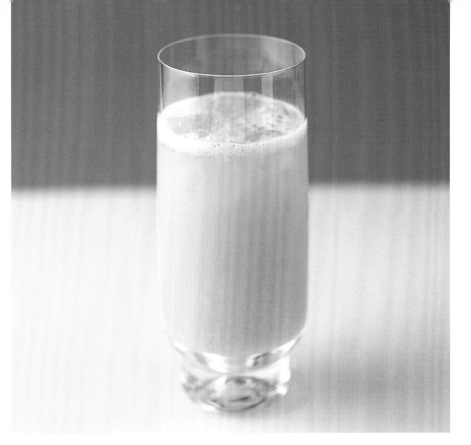

# 345

## broccoli, parsnip + apple
juice

SERVES 1

**150 g (5½ oz) broccoli**
**50 g (1¾ oz) parsnip**
**50 g (1¾ oz) apple**
**2–3 ice cubes**

Trim the broccoli. Peel the parsnip and remove the stalk from the apple.

Juice the prepared ingredients together.

Transfer the juice to a blender or food processor, add the ice cubes and blend to make a creamy juice.

Pour the juice into a glass and serve immediately.

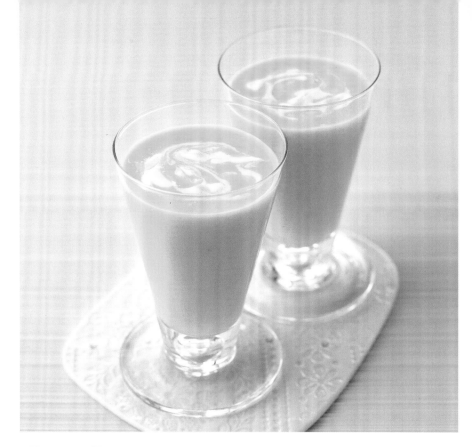

# 346

## peach + orange smoothie

SERVES 2

**200 g (7 oz) canned peaches in natural juice**

**75 ml (2½ fl oz) peach or apricot yogurt, plus extra to decorate**

**100 ml (3½ fl oz) fresh orange juice**

**1 teaspoon clear honey (optional)**

**ice cubes (optional)**

Drain the peaches and use the juice in another recipe.

Put the peaches in a blender or smoothie maker, add the yogurt, orange juice and honey, if using, and blend until smooth.

Pour the smoothie over ice cubes, if using, in glasses, top with a swirl of extra yogurt and serve immediately.

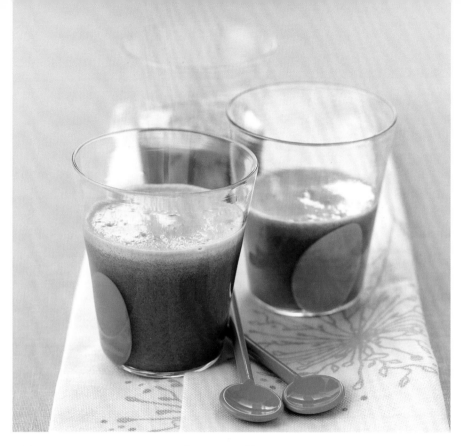

# 347

## broccoli, spinach + apple
juice

SERVES 1

**150 g (5½ oz) broccoli**

**150 g (5½ oz) spinach**

**2 apples**

**2–3 ice cubes**

Trim the broccoli and rinse the spinach. Remove the stalks from the apples.

Juice the apples with the spinach and broccoli, alternating the spinach leaves with the other ingredients so that the spinach leaves do not clog the machine.

Transfer the juice to a blender or food processor, add the ice cubes and blend briefly.

Pour the juice into a glass and serve immediately.

# 348

## passionfruit + lemon grass infusion

SERVES 1

**1 lemon grass stalk**
**200 ml (7 fl oz) boiling water**
**2 passionfruits**
**juice of 1 lime**
**2 teaspoons clear honey**

Cut the lemon grass stalk in half lengthways, then finely chop one of the halves. Put in a small bowl and pour over the measured boiling water. Leave to infuse for 3–4 minutes.

Halve the passionfruits and scoop out the seeds and pulp into a tea strainer set over a cup. Press the pulp with the back of a teaspoon to extract the juice.

Add the lime juice to the cup and strain in the lemon grass infusion through the strainer. Stir in the honey, add the halved lemon grass stalk as a stirrer and serve hot.

Both passionfruits and lemon grass have antiseptic properties.

# 349

## mango, melon + orange juice

SERVES 1

**2 oranges**
**1 mango**
**½ galia melon**
**2 ice cubes**

Peel the oranges and then juice.

Peel and stone the mango, then roughly chop the flesh. Peel the melon as close to the skin as possible and deseed, then roughly chop the flesh.

Put the mango and melon flesh in a blender or smoothie maker and blend until smooth. Add the orange juice and ice cubes, then blend again until smooth.

Pour the juice into a glass and serve immediately.

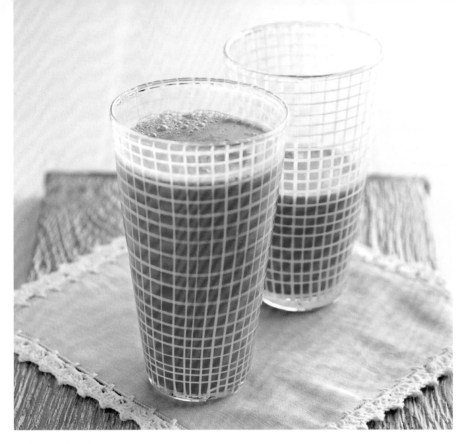

# 350

## cranberry + carrot juice

SERVES 1

**2 carrots**

**1 orange**

**225 g (8 oz) cranberries**

Take the tops off the carrots and then scrub. Peel the orange.

Juice all the ingredients together.

Pour the juice into a glass and serve immediately.

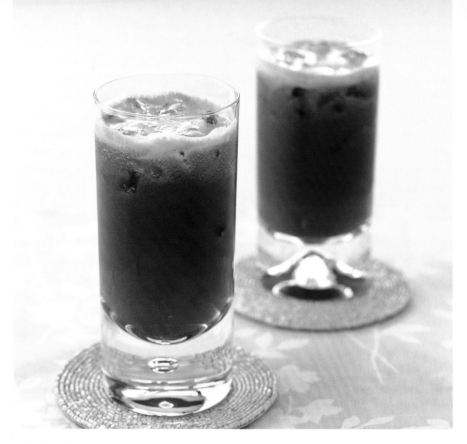

# 351

## herbed broccoli + kale juice

**SERVES 1**

**100 g (3½ oz) broccoli**
**100 g (3½ oz) kale**
**50 g (1¾ oz) celery**
**200 g (7 oz) apples**
**25 g (1 oz) parsley**
**ice cubes**

Trim the broccoli. Cut any really woody stalks off the kale. Peel away any stringy bits from the celery. Remove the stalks from the apples.

Juice the prepared ingredients with the parsley.

Pour the juice over ice cubes in a glass and serve immediately.

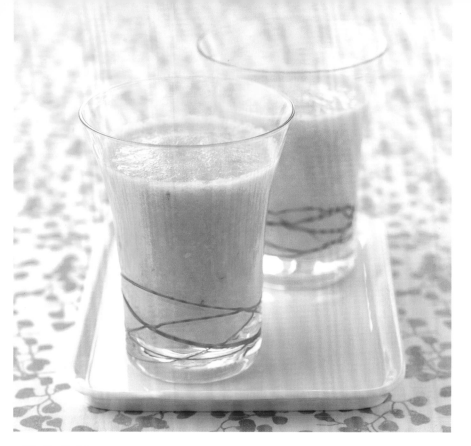

# 352

## mandarin + lychee frappé

SERVES 1

**100 g (3½ oz) canned mandarin oranges in natural juice**

**50 g (1¾ oz) canned lychees in natural juice**

**ice cubes**

Put the mandarin oranges and lychees with the juices from the cans into a blender or smoothie maker, add the ice cubes and blend briefly.

Pour the frappé into a glass and serve immediately.

# 353

## passionfruit, mango + lime smoothie

SERVES 4

**1 lime**
**2 large mangoes**
**5 passionfruits**
**225 g (8 oz) natural yogurt**
**2 handfuls of ice cubes**

Peel and then juice the lime. Peel and stone the mangoes, then roughly chop the flesh.

Transfer the lime juice to a blender or smoothie maker. Halve the passionfruits, scoop out the seeds and pulp and add all but 1 tablespoon to the blender or smoothie maker with the mangoes, yogurt and ice cubes, then blend until smooth.

Pour the smoothie into glasses, decorate with the reserved passionfruit pulp and seeds and serve immediately.

# 354

## kale, melon + pear juice

SERVES 1

**100 g (3½ oz) kale**
**1 pear**
**½ cantaloupe melon**
**½ lime**
**¼ cucumber**

Cut any really woody stalks off the kale. Remove the stalk from the pear. Peel the melon as close to the skin as possible and deseed, then roughly chop.

Juice the kale, pear and melon with the unpeeled lime half and cucumber.

Pour the juice into a glass and serve immediately.

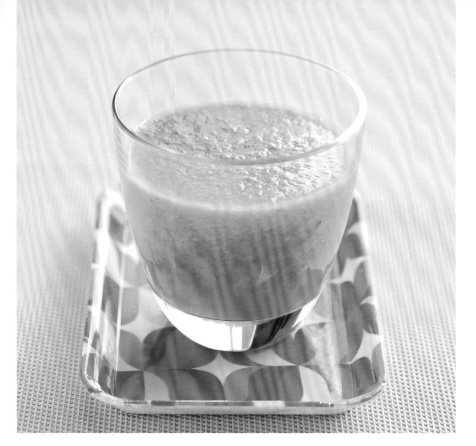

# 355

## blueberry + pomegranate
juice

SERVES 1

**2 pomegranates**

**1 lemon**

**200 g (7 oz) blueberries**

Remove the seeds from the pomegranate by cutting the fruit in half, then holding the halved fruit over a bowl and hitting the skin with a wooden spoon so that the seeds fall into the bowl. Peel the lemon.

Juice all the ingredients together.

Pour the juice into a glass and serve immediately.

# 356

## raspberry, grape + apricot juice

SERVES 1

**1 apricot**

**1 carrot**

**200 g (7 oz) raspberries, plus extra to decorate**

**12 red seedless grapes**

Halve and stone the apricot. Take the top off the carrot and then scrub.

Juice all the ingredients together.

Pour the juice into a glass, decorate with a few raspberries and serve immediately.

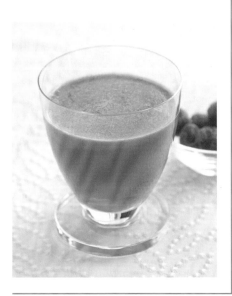

# 357

## cherry + flax seed smoothie

SERVES 1

**150 g (5½ oz) sweet dark cherries**

**¼ pineapple**

**100 ml (3½ fl oz) coconut water**

**1 teaspoon flax seeds**

Stone the cherries. Cut the skin off the pineapple and remove the core if very tough, then roughly chop.

Put all ingredients in a blender or smoothie maker and blend until smooth.

Pour the smoothie into a glass and serve immediately.

# 358

## next time...

Swap the cherries for 150 g (5½ oz) blueberries and the flax seeds for 1 teaspoon chia seeds, then blend with the pineapple and coconut water until smooth.

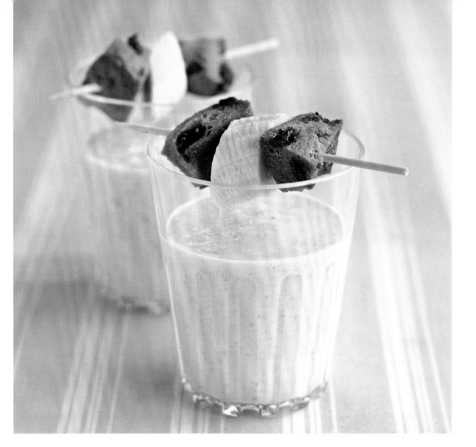

# 359

## banana + maple syrup
### smoothie

SERVES 2

**2 bananas, plus extra slices to decorate**

**300 ml (10 fl oz) milk**

**4 tablespoons natural fromage frais**

**3 tablespoons maple syrup**

**50 g (1¾ oz) hot oat cereal**

**malt loaf chunks, to decorate**

Peel the bananas, then roughly chop. Put in a blender or smoothie maker, add the milk, fromage frais and maple syrup and blend until smooth. Add the oat cereal and blend again to thicken.

Pour the smoothie into glasses. To decorate, arrange banana slices and chunks of malt loaf on cocktail sticks and balance them across the top of the glasses. Serve immediately.

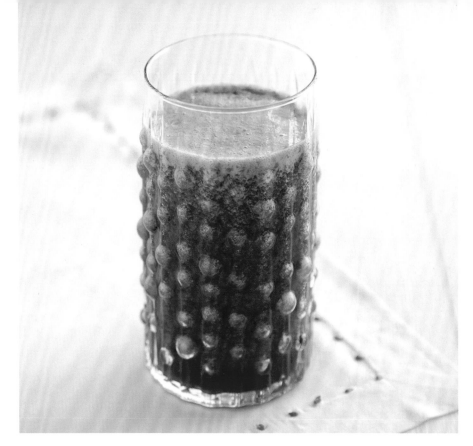

# 360

## plum, peach + apricot
juice

**SERVES 1**

**4 plums**

**3 peaches**

**2 apricots**

**1 carrot**

**ice cubes**

Halve and stone the plums, peaches and apricots. Take the top off the carrot and then scrub.

Juice all the prepared ingredients together.

Pour the juice over ice cubes in a glass and serve immediately.

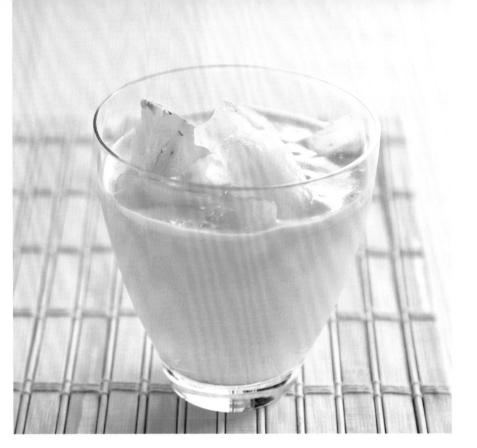

# 361

## pineapple + coconut water
juice

SERVES 1

**400 g (14 oz) pineapple, plus an extra small wedge to decorate**

**200 ml (7 fl oz) coconut water**

**ice cubes**

Cut the skin off the pineapple and remove the core if very tough, then roughly chop the flesh.

Juice the pineapple, then stir in the coconut water.

Pour the juice over ice cubes in a glass, decorate with a small pineapple wedge and serve immediately.

233

# 362

## nectarine + raspberry yogurt ice

SERVES 2

**3 nectarines**
**175 g (6 oz) raspberries**
**150 g (5½ oz) natural yogurt**
**handful of ice cubes**

Halve and stone the nectarines. Put in a blender or smoothie maker with the raspberries and blend until smooth.

Add the yogurt and blend again, then add the ice cubes and blend until finely crushed and the mixture thickens.

Pour the mixture into 2 chilled glasses, decorate with cocktail umbrellas, if liked, and serve immediately.

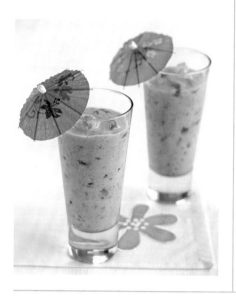

# 363

## grape, beetroot + plum juice

SERVES 1

**2 small plums, plus extra wedges to decorate**
**2 small beetroots**
**100 g (3½ oz) red seedless grapes**
**ice cubes**

Halve and stone the plums. Trim the beetroot and then scrub or peel.

Juice the prepared ingredients with the grapes.

Pour the juice over ice cubes in a glass, decorate with plum wedges and serve immediately.

tip

This juice is high in folate from the beetroot.

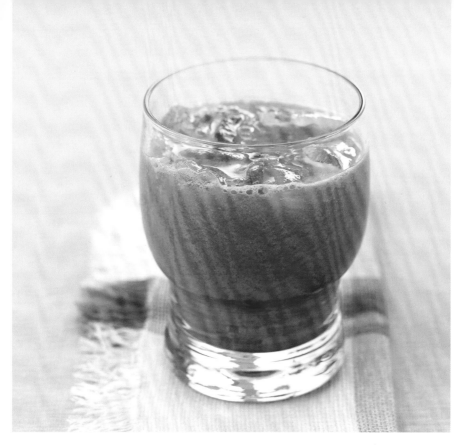

## 364

### watermelon + raspberry
juice

SERVES 1

**300 g (10½ oz) watermelon**
**125 g (4½ oz) raspberries**
**2–3 ice cubes**

Peel the melon as close to the skin as possible and deseed, then roughly chop the flesh.

Juice the melon and raspberries together.

Pour the juice into a glass, add the ice cubes and serve immediately.

## 365
next time...

For a tangy alternative, juice the watermelon with 2 oranges, peeled, in place of the raspberries.

**235**

# index

# picture credits

Additional picture credits:

**Octopus Publishing Group** Vanessa Davies 144, 161, 177, 203; Janine Hosegood 6a, 6b, 7, 8a, 8b, 28, 65, 83; Lis Parsons 10, 11, 12, 13, 14, 15, 18, 19, 20, 22, 25, 27, 29, 33, 34, 36, 37, 38, 39, 40, 42, 45, 47, 49, 54, 55, 56, 61, 63, 64, 66, 68, 69, 70, 71, 72, 75, 78, 81, 82, 85, 86, 87, 91, 92, 95, 96, 97, 103, 104, 106, 108, 109, 112, 114, 115, 117, 118, 119, 124, 125, 126, 128, 129, 130, 131, 132, 134, 135, 137, 138, 142, 143, 145, 146, 147, 151, 152, 154, 155, 158, 159, 160, 162, 163, 166, 168, 169, 172, 173, 174, 175, 176, 178, 179, 180, 181, 183, 184, 185, 186, 187, 190, 191, 192, 193, 194, 195, 196, 197, 198, 199, 200, 201, 202, 208, 209, 211, 213, 214, 215, 216, 217, 218, 219, 220, 221, 222, 223, 225, 226, 227, 229, 230, 232, 233, 235; Gareth Sambidge 32, 41, 48, 60, 79, 80, 89, 90; William Shaw 139.

# acknowledgements

**Publishing Director:** Stephanie Jackson
**Editor:** Natalie Bradley
**Contributor:** Angela Dowden
**Copy-editor:** Jo Richardson
**Proofreader:** Jane Birch
**Indexer:** Isobel McLean

**Senior Designer:** Jaz Bahra
**Design & Art Direction:** Geoff Fennell
**Special Photography:** William Shaw
**Home Economist:** Sara Lewis
**Prop Stylist:** Kim Sullivan
**Production Controller:** Meskerem Berhane